HERBS:

Partners in Life

HERBS:
Partners in Life

*Healing, Gardening, and Cooking
with Wild Plants*

Adele G. Dawson

With a Foreword by Rosemary Gladstar

Illustrated by Robin Rothman

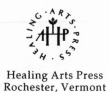

Healing Arts Press
Rochester, Vermont

Healing Arts Press
One Park Street
Rochester, Vermont 05767
www.InnerTraditions.com

Healing Arts Press is a division of Inner Traditions International

*Note to the reader: This book is intended as an informational guide. The remedies,
approaches, and techniques described herein are meant to supplement, and not to be a
substitute for, professional medical care or treatment. They should not be used to treat
a serious ailment without prior consultation with a qualified health care professional.*

Library of Congress Cataloging-in-Publication Data

Dawson, Adele Godchaux.
    Herbs : partners in life : healing, gardening, and cooking with wild plants /
    Adele G. Dawson.
        p. cm.
    Includes bibliographical references (p.).
    ISBN 0-89281-934-0 (alk. paper)
    1. Herbs. 2. Herbs—Therapeutic use. 3. Cookery (Herbs) 4.Herbs— Folklore.
    5. Herb gardening. I. Title.

SB351 .H5 D39 2000
635'.7—dc21

                                                                    00-040913

Printed and bound in the United States

10 9 8 7 6 5 4 3 2 1

This book was typeset in Palatino

Contents

PART II

Foreword

Herbs: Partners in Life is one of the great herbal treasures of our time. Tucked throughout every page is the wisdom and wit of nine decades of an extraordinary life. Adele was considered by all who met her to be a grand human being. In her home state of Vermont, she was often referred to as a "state treasure." Her home was certainly a mecca, the Grand Central Station of Marshfield. Worldwide travelers, casual visitors, and friends would stop by to chat with this wise old elder and stroll in her marvelous unruly herb gardens. Having heard of her, visitors whom she'd never met would stop by on a whim and were soon added to her ever-expanding circle of friends.

I met Adele during my first year in Vermont. I barely survived my first winter and was seriously questioning why any self-respecting herbalists would chose to live in a place where winter ruled for six months of the year. Having just moved from a perfect zone 8 in northern

California to a rocky granite outcrop only two planting zones away from the arctic cap, I had a right to doubt my sanity. I might have packed up and gone home had not Adele stopped by to visit. In true plant lover's style, she brought several hardy herb plants from her garden to my unpromising newly tilled soil and warmly invited me for tea at her "tea house." Her welcome won my heart. Watching the way that this tiny spritelike woman walked through the gardens, the way she spoke to the plants, the way they spoke back to her, and the sparkle in her eyes, I recognized that I was in the presence of a great herbal elder. That great spirit of hers, disguised in the tiny frame of an old woman, fairly danced around me, and drew me in, forever quelling any doubts I had as to what I was doing in Vermont. We rapidly became friends and in the ensuing years she was a mentor and teacher to me. Along with many opportunities to be with her, I had the good fortune to be her "chauffeur," driving her to the many herb events and gatherings of which she was always the star. What a treat for me! On those long rides, I was not only entertained by her endless stories, but also steeped in the rich lore of plants.

Lucky for me, Adele lived nearby, just over the hill as the crow flies. Nestled in the small village of Marshfield in the Northeast Kingdom of Vermont, her large rambling farmhouse was surrounded by a mostly untamed garden that ran wildly up the hillside. Lush with herbs, wildflowers, and useful weeds, her garden was reflective of the free spirit of its owner. Directly next to the house flowed one of Vermont's longest waterfalls. It was spectacular. Here, in a setting that was as paradisial as any one could imagine, Adele worked her charm on a community of people.

I was constantly amazed at Adele's accomplishments and interests. She had lived through many chapters in her nine decades of life. I knew her as an herbalist, extraordinary gardener, and healer. But others knew her as an artist, a writer, a political activist, and a homemaker. As an activist and ecologist, she lobbied endlessly for the environment and often spoke out for better agricultural practices and the safeguarding of wildlands and wetlands. She'd raised a family of six children. Sometime in her latter years, she took up yoga and mediation. She loved to travel and enjoyed "off the beaten path" adventures well into her nineties. Truthfully, I'm not sure there wasn't much that was good in the world that Adele wasn't ready to experience, and she filled whatever circle she was in with her stories, laughter, political discussions, and endless observations on the many interests she had acquired in her long rich

life. Truly she embodied the élan vital, the essence of life, and passed
iiòalong freely—and often those with whom she shared her zest were
decades younger.

Sometimes when I'm teaching my herb classes, I find myself quoting
Adele. "So long as they think we're crazy, we're safe" were her funny
but wise words to menopausal women. People often asked her about
her secret to long life, and she knew they were waiting for a secret
herbal tonic or favorite dietary suggestions. Little did they know that
Adele was a moderation guru. "Everything in moderation," she would
say as she ate and drank whatever she chose. Her other secret to long
life? "One must be very careful who one chooses as one's parents."

When she passed away at the ripe age of ninety-four, quickly and
quite suddenly at her home, along with the to-be-expected sadness and
grief we all felt was the shared feeling of surprise. I don't think any of
us ever expected Adele to die. Her passing was another teaching to us.
Adele was finishing up her latest work, a cookbook of her favorite herbal
recipes. She was inviting friends over every few days to sample her
latest recipes. I'd eaten lunch with her a few days earlier. The food was
delicious and she was in great spirits. Later in the week, she invited a
few friends over for breakfast. She rose early, walked the mile or two
to the local post office, mailed her membership fee to the Northeast
Herb Association, an organization that she had helped found a few
years earlier, and returned home to fix breakfast for her friends. The
rest of the story may be part of how legends grow, but this is the way
the story was told. Adele sat down at the table with her friends and as
they began breakfast a great white owl flew to a tree outside the window. Adele took a few deep breaths and quietly passed away or, perhaps, in accordance with legends, flew away with the spirit of Artemis's
sacred bird.

This book, the only major compilation of her wisdom, is a treasure
and gift to us and should be accounted among the great herb books of
the twentieth century. Adele's spirit—her love, kindness, and compas-
sion—fills every page. I was fortunate to know Adele in person. We are
all fortunate that she left her legacy to us in this book.

Rosemary Gladstar
East Barre, Vermont
20 June 2000

Preface

To us in the modern world who understand the process which causes the cosmic phenomena of the seasons to follow each other inevitably, it may seem that primitive man's attempt to insure the arrival of spring by dressing in leaves and acting out the return of verdure, of making an effigy of winter and "killing" it to make way for new vegetation, was foolish indeed. Yet, when we begin to think about the change of seasons, we see that we are still tied closely to them, physically and psychically. A rational explanation does not eliminate the mystic meaning. We are different people in each season with different needs for food, amount of rest, and sleep.

Our energies vary: we are extrovert, introvert, far more affected by moon-rise and moon-set than we may realize. If we analyze the qualities of each season, we see that we, too, act out the drama of birth, growth, maturity, decay, and rebirth every day of our lives.

By attuning to the seasons in our relationship with herbs which have been given to us "for meat and medicine" we will get closer to them and to ourselves.

When William Wordsworth wrote, in 1807, "The world is too much with us," it was a prophetic statement more pertinent today than it was then. Our gardens, as well as the herbs that grow in them, may be a mini-universe in which over-stressed bodies and souls can retreat from the relentless bombardment of information (and information is not the same as knowledge) which penetrates our homes, cars, planes, airports, and department stores.

In the peace and quiet of a garden we can choose our own cosmology, fitted gently to our belief system. In ancient Egypt and China, three separate cosmologies existed side by side—three different ways of seeing the universe. Whether we consider this contradictory or complementary may be a measure of minds.

The way we understand our garden, the life in it, is the way we understand ourself. We both date back millions of years, not in our present forms, although we still have vestiges of ancient victories and defeats. The plants of this year's garden have the resonance of the past in every thrusting root, every stem that leans into or resists a breeze, every blossom that opens or closes on signal from the sun. Thousands of years ago, fungi, lichens, moss, ferns grew beneath our basil, dill, sage; beneath roses, violets, lilies.

Underneath our 20th century brain, the neocortex, lurks the limbic system which we share with all mammals, and beneath this is our old reptilian brain made up of the hypothalmus and basal ganglia.

Imprints of the past in both garden and self affect health and wisdom. The basic function of past lives was survival. The abilities to adapt and to establish companionate relationships are due to trail and error over the centuries.

Native Americans speak of "all our relations." They refer to the deer, the bear, the eagle, the serpent, and the butterfly; to trees, rivers, and mountains.

"All our relations" may not be merely a metaphoric way of describing other species that share the earth with us. Modern science has established that our "first language," a pre-natal one made up of only four nucleotides, is quite similar in every form of life. It consists of a simple manual of instructions, a how-to guide that causes each species to resemble its parents. The mouse child will be a mouse, the elephant child an elephant. A carrot seed will produce a carrot, a tarragon seed will become a tarragon plant.

In contemporary life it is important for gardeners to remind themselves that science did not develop these instructions for all species. It only discovered that they existed. The Great Spirit did not give instructions to one species for the benefit of another. Evolution can continue only if organisms maintain an enormous array of genetic diversity.

Symbols go back to the beginning of mankind. The double helix that led to the discovery of DNA existed in every part of the world. The symbol of two snakes coiled around a central staff with two bird wings on top is found in many cultures—in Egypt, India, Mexico, Greece. In each place it comes from inherited traditional lore. But the meaning of the symbols—two basic opposites, chtonic force and higher consciousness—is always the same.

A garden, small or large, like a nuclear or extended family, gives us a protected, friendly place to grow—not only to grow herbs in a way compatible with nature, but to grow in our own psychic awareness, to cultivate our potential for being sensitive and responsible citizens of the planet and grateful caretakers of our inherited treasures.

Grow slender weeds
Absorb energy
from the cosmos
so you might heal.

C. DAVID SINEX

Introduction

An introduction to her book requires of the author two things: She has written the book and she has read it. In the first capacity she is the architect, in the second the guide.

As a guide, I would like to point out the paths leading to the main structure. Part I deals with the philosophy of using herbs for food, drink and medicine, where they are found, gathered, or purchased, how they are stored and used. This section also includes an illustrated introduction to botanical terms that describe herbs, and a short who's who of herbalists referred to in the text.

In Part II we plant, gather, preserve, smell, enjoy, eat, drink, and prescribe herbs. Monographs of more than seventy genera are described and illustrated. These are divided into four groups which will be found at the end of the four seasonal chapters on spring, summer, autumn, and winter, sections reinforced with alchemy, astrology, botany, biochemistry, folklore, history, literature, and modern life.

The discussions of specific herbs are headed by the common, general name of the herb (Agrimony in the example below). Below it, on the left, are common names given to herb species answering to the general name; folk or local names of the same species are given in quotes and parentheses. On the right, in italics, are corresponding Latin names of the species (*Agrimonia eupatoria* L.), and the name of the family of plants to which the species belongs (*ROSACEAE*). Letters following the Latin species name are the initial letter or letters of the name of the botanist who first described the species—most often the eighteenth-century botanist, Linnaeus (L.).

AGRIMONY

AGRIMONY   *Agrimonia eupatoria L.*
("COCKLEBURR," "STICKLEWORT")
                                                  ROSACEAE

The botanical name usually carries a bit of history. In this case, *Agrimonia* comes from the Greek word "argemone" which means healing to the eyes. *Eupatoria* honors Mithridates, Eupator of Pontus, an ancient king noted for his extensive herb garden and herbal remedies. The first word is always the genus, the second the species.

In the appendix are alphabetical lists of the herbs described in the book, a glossary of the words used to describe the medicinal action of individual herbs; a check-list of vitamins and their actions on the human system; bibliographies according to subject; and a source list of seeds, plants and botanicals.

At this point your guide leaves you—bon voyage.

PART I

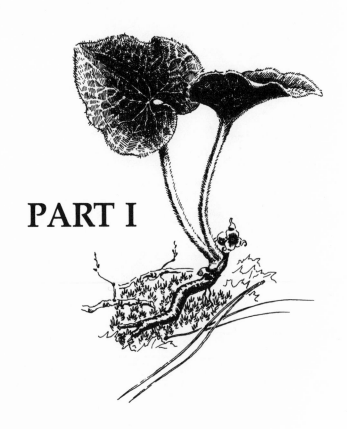

I

Why Should We
Use Herbs?

In 1816 Thomas Greene wrote in his *Universal Herbal*, "Nature has in this country, as well as in all others, provided in the herbs of its own growth the remedies for the several diseases to which it is most subject."

The woods and fields of New England are a treasure house of wild herbs, natural and effective remedies for the common imbalances that sometimes plague us as a result of fatigue, infection, or accident. Damp stream-beds are rimmed with large green rounds of coltsfoot leaves and the rich humus-carpeted woods nurture beds of wild leeks, blue cohosh, and goldthread. A walk across any abandoned meadow will yield a therapeutic bouquet of gold-flowered St. John's-wort and tall mullein spikes. Fern-like tansy and white, sometimes pink, flowered yarrow defy the encroaching crabgrass. Ditch edges in August host fluffy white spikes of flowering boneset, and along rutted country roads monarch butterflies feed on purple clusters of milkweed blossoms. Dozens of "garden herbs" can be grown easily in our backyards—hardy perennials, whose welcome appearance each springs is, happily, more dependent on sunshine and good drainage than the expertise of even a pale green thumb. Both wild and cultivated herbs are dual-purpose plants, delicious and economical food and drink as well as safe and proven remedies.

In the 19th century the scientific establishment was so enchanted with bacteriology that its attention was focused on the external rather than the internal cause of disease. Unfortunately this bias is prevalent today, resulting in the treatment of the symptom rather than the cause. Chinese medicine, with three thousand years of philosophical pondering behind it, never wandered into this cul-de-sac. It is directed toward maintaining the balance and harmony of the body as the best prevention of disease. In the "Huang Ti Nei Ching Su Wen" (*The Yellow Emperor's Classic of Internal Medicine*), the legendary Emperor of 2500 B.C. asked his physician, "What constitutes a healthy person?" To which Chi Po answered, "A healthy and well-balanced person is not affected by disease."

This is the basic philosophy today of herbalists who use vegetable medicines to maintain a balance of the body and a serenity of the mind, enabling each to provide its own cure. We define health as that mental, physical, and spiritual development which provides for each of us a complete life, satisfying to ourselves and helpful to others. There is no standard blueprint for us to use; each good life must be "owner-built" because we all enter the world with unique characteristics, a medley of genetic inheritance and prenatal influence. We carry this predetermined equipment with us into adulthood, and its appraisal and programming is part of our adult responsibility. This includes acceptance of the untidy fact that our bodies vary in efficiency of workmanship as well as in beauty of design. These differences must be faced serenely when we seek to identify a malfunction for purposes of prevention or cure. We must know our own strengths and weaknesses and learn to be sensitive to the signals our body uses to alert us to its needs. "Symptoms," often mistaken for disease, are manifestations which the body uses to alert us to the fact that something is wrong; certain cells or organs are either not getting what they need to function properly or are being subjected to something that is bad for them.

Paracelsus, Swiss physician and alchemist born about 1493 as Phillippus Aureolus Theophrastus Bombastus von Hohenheim, said, "He who wants to know man must look upon him as a whole and not a patched up piece of work. If he finds a part of the human body diseased, he must look for the causes that produce the disease and not merely treat the external effects."

The causes of disease are often multiple, sometimes indirect; they may lurk behind little-noticed dangers of short-sighted or profit-motivated technology. Here is a check-list of some common background causes of poor health:

1. Excessive (constant) use of "junk foods"
   a. Foods with artificial coloring and/or artificial flavoring
   b. Foods with preservatives (for longer "shelf-life" but possibly shorter human life)
   c. Package foods that substitute synthetic for natural food
2. Fast foods, eaten in a hurry or in an atmosphere lacking in serenity and visual pleasure
3. Continued tension
4. Over-exposure to artificial light
5. Lack of exposure to natural light, not necessarily sunlight
6. Continued fatigue
7. Excessive exposure (daily) to pollutants:
   a. Chemical
   b. Mineral
   c. Radioactive
   d. Noise
   e. Air-borne
8. Dissatisfaction with:
   a. Job
   b. Social life and social situation
   c. Family situation
9. Lack of opportunity for:
   a. Exercise
   b. Continuing education
   c. Creative leisure-time interests
   d. Service to others (community service, sharing of abilities)
10. Excessive use of:
    a. Cigarettes
    b. Stimulants and depressants
    c. Pills

Scanning this list, you may find an unobtrusive cause of stress in your body which is producing symptoms whose cause you may not have traced. Exposure to virus and bacterial infection is not included in the list because the "healthy and well-balanced person," as Chi Po suggested to the Emperor, is seldom affected by disease.

Thousands of medicinal herbs exist from which over half the drugs sold in pharmacies, on prescription and as proprietary medicine, are derived. Coeburn Produce Company Inc., of Virginia, in its 1975 brochure lists 118 herb leaves, roots, and barks that it buys to sell to pharmaceutical houses. Forty-three of these are in regular demand, and nineteen are especially needed. This company has been buying from gatherers of wild herbs since 1891.

Those of us who are ready to take more responsibility for our own health realize that herbal remedies prepared at home have three distinct advantages over commercially-formulated drugs. Herbs are selected which respond to the need of a person, not a disease. We all know from actual experience in our own families that disease affects each one of us differently, according to our area of weakness and body chemistry. It is common sense to use a remedy compounded to meet an individual need.

Another plus for our own herbal preparations is that we use the herbs that grow in the same environment in which we live; we share the same climate, seasons, air, soil, and water. Calcium, iron, iodine, magnesium, potassium, phosphorus, and sodium, as well as the trace minerals copper, manganese, and zinc exist in plants. Those plants that grow in our own environment will contain the substances we need to maintain health.

Hippocrates, called the Father of Medicine, said, "Look to the country and to the season before deciding on treatment."

One last advantage to making our own herbal medicine, tea, poultice, or salve: We use the herb with its chemical constituents intact, exactly as it occurs in nature. The pharmaceutical companies extract what they believe to be the "active ingredient" and mix it in a laboratory with synthetic substances. This is why commercially prepared drugs often have a side effect which may surface as a rash, increased heart beat, breathing difficulty, or drowsiness.

The average testing time for new pharmaceutical products is a few years, hardly sufficient to measure long-term effects. Plants that we use today, in their natural state, have been used for 60,000 years, since the time of Neanderthal man. In the ancient burials at Shanidar, near

Baghdad, flowering plants were found, many of which still grow in the same area around Iraq and are known to be astringents, diuretics (useful to increase the flow of urine), emetics, pain relievers, and stimulants.

Our "materia medica" in this book will be confined to some seventy herbs, wild and cultivated. The herbs have been chosen because all are completely harmless even if used without accurate measurements, because they are common to many localities throughout the country, and because they are easy to recognize by shape, scent, and growing habit. Last but not least, they were selected because they alleviate most of the common health problems that confront us. Many of these herbs have more than one use, and all of them have been used by the author for half a century.

The maladies for which these herbs are helpful include:

allergies	indigestion
arthritis	insomnia
asthma	menstrual problems
bee stings	muscular pains
blood pressure	poison ivy
boils	rheumatism
bronchitis	sciatica
colds	sinus
colic	splinters
constipation	sunburn
coughs	tension
cuts	varicose veins
cystitis	warts
diarrhea	worms
fatigue	wounds
headaches	

Remember that the "x" ingredient in herbal medicine, as in all medicine, is common sense. As you read this book you will see that there is always more than one herb having certain medical properties. When you select herbs to meet one of the above problems you must also consider your own individual needs. To do this it is sensible to analyze your own constitution and life-style. For example: It is winter; you have a job that uses up nervous as well as physical energy; your food at lunch consists of whatever is available near your place of work; you catch cold; the cold goes into bronchitis. You must choose from among several herbs that are specific for bronchitis. Which do you use and what herbs do you combine with them? Obviously you will choose some herbs that have nutritive value, that are soothing to the nerves and will improve circulation. This is what we mean by common sense in herbal medicine.

Cotton Mather (1663–1728), better known for his sermons than for his pharmacopeia, extolled the virtues of many wild herbs as well as garden plants. "It would be," he said, "a 'laudable thing' for gentlewomen to keep in their closets a number of harmless and useful herbs to help their neighbors if they needed them." This advice is just as sound, and humane, today as it was in 1700 when Pastor Mather (son of Increase) delivered his lengthy sermons amid a minty aroma of "Bible leaf" or costmary (*Balsamita major*) as devout Christians stayed awake by chewing the serrated leaves, kept conveniently as bookmarks in their Bibles.

II

Identification of Herbs

Herbs, like other plants, may be identified by the formation and other characteristics of their roots, stems, leaves, and flowers. Herbalists and botanists have terms of their own to describe characteristics of the plants they study and use. In this chapter a number of important terms are introduced, many of which will be used in the chapters that follow.

ROOTS

Many herbs have enlarged roots with distinctive shapes. Four common root forms are pictured on the following page: taproot, napiform (turnip-shaped), fusiform (spindle-shaped), and tuberous. The figure also shows an underground stem or rhizome.

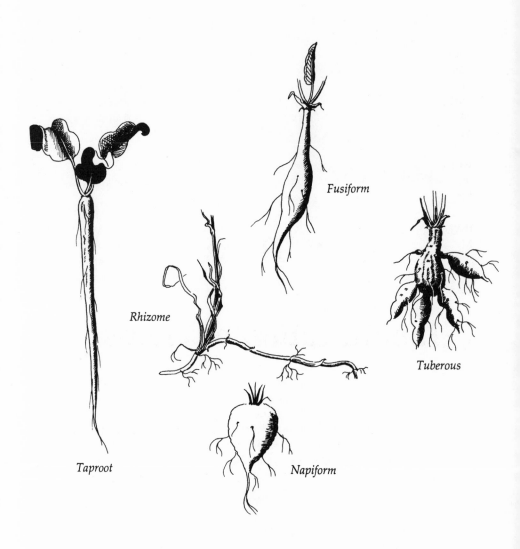

Fusiform

Rhizome

Tuberous

Taproot

Napiform

Rhizome and root formation

STEMS

There are two basic types of stems and branches: those that appear above ground, and those that do not. Plants whose stem and branches rise above the ground are said to have a "true" stem, or, in botany, to be "caulescent." In temperate climates, most herbs are caulescent. Plants with stems that are not visible above ground are called stemless or "acaulescent." You will easily recognize crocus, bloodroot and violets as being acaulescent.

Some herbs have prostrate underground stems called "rhizomes," which spread below ground, at intervals putting down roots and sending up leaves and flowers. Couch grass and the clovers are examples of herbs having rhizomes (see figure on page 12).

The way in which stems and branches of caulescent plants arrange themselves on the ground offers a useful clue for identifying the plant. Most herbs have erect stems. Four other kinds of stem arrangement are:

1. *Diffuse* (stems spread loosely over the ground in all directions);
2. *Declined* (stems bend to one side);
3. *Decumbent* (stems lie flat on the ground as if not strong enough to support the weight of the plant);
4. *Prostrate or Procumbent* (stems are strong, but lie along the ground);
5. *Creeping or repent* (stems lie on ground, putting down new roots as they grow horizontally).

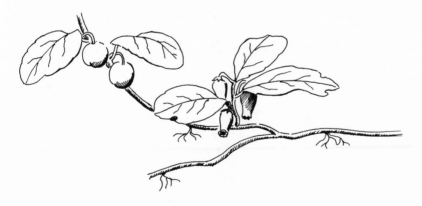

Repent or creeping stem

13

LEAVES

The principal part of a leaf is usually referred to as the "blade." Other leaf parts are shown in the figure. "Stipules" are small leaflike appendages attached to the petiole where it joins the plant stem (that is, at the "axil").

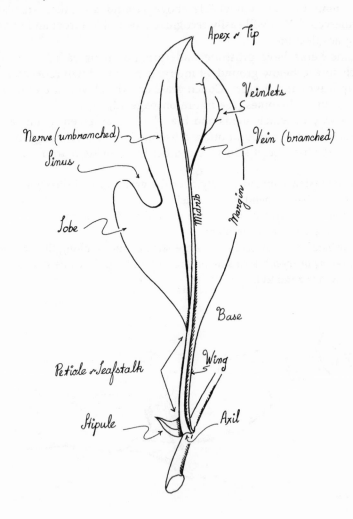

Parts of a leaf

Venation

The arrangement of veins on a leaf blade may help to identify the plant that bears the leaf. Venation may be "netted" (also called "reticulated") or "nerved" (also called "parallel"). Both are pictured.

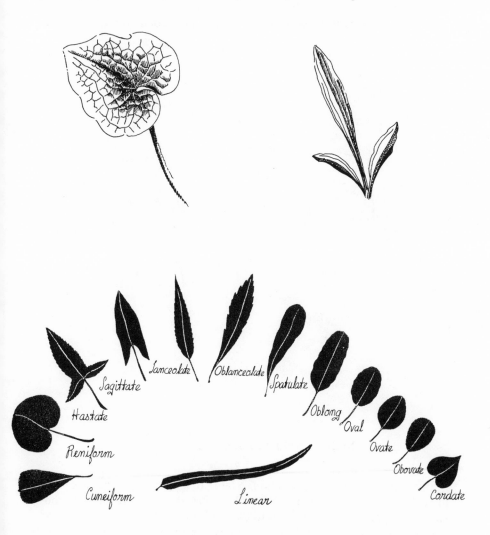

Leaf shapes

Leaf Shapes

Leaf shapes, how leaves are arranged on the stem, and how they are attached to the stem, are three highly individual characteristics of plant species. The silhouette drawing of leaf shapes shows thirteen common shapes.

In addition, leaves of various shapes may be "lobed" or "cleft" as in the next figure.

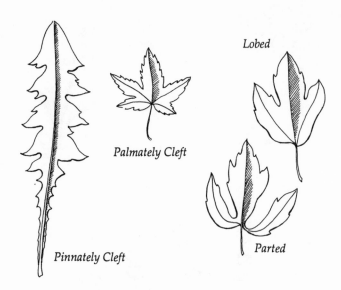

Lobed

Palmately Cleft

Pinnately Cleft

Parted

More leaf shapes

Simple and Compound Leaves

In another important distinction, related to leaf shape, leaves are said to be "simple" or "compound." Simple leaves are attached singly to the stem. Compound leaves are subdivided around the leaf midrib, consisting of several smaller "leaflets," as shown in the figure on page 17.

The arrangement of leaflets on the midrib of a compound leaf may be "pinnate" (feather-like) or "palmate" (leaflets radiate from a center), as in the drawing.

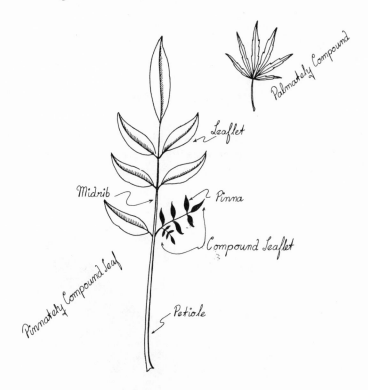

Compound leaves and their parts

LEAF TIPS

The tip or free end of a leaf may also have a distinctive shape. Eight terms used to describe leaf end-shapes are:

1. *Pointed* (said of leaves ending in a pronounced, sharp point);
2. *Acute* (not so sharply point, but ending in an acute angle);

3. *Obtuse* (ending in a blunt point);
4. *Truncate* (square-tipped);
5. *Retuse* (slightly indented, rounded tip);
6. *Emarginate* (notched at the end);
7. *Cuspidate* (having a sharp and rigid point);
8. *Mucronate* (abruptly tipped with a small, sharp point).

LEAF MARGIN TYPES

The margin or edge of the leaf blade varies widely among plant species and can be an important factor in identification. The schematic drawing shows ten possibilities for margin formation.

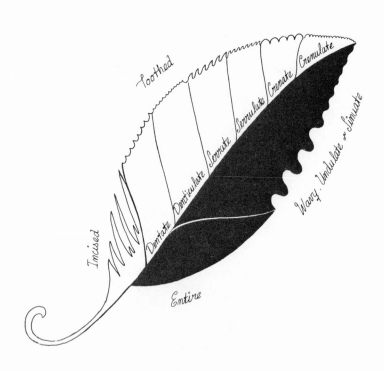

Common leaf margin types

Leaf Arrangement and Attachment

Leaves may be arranged on the stem "opposite" one another, like the two at the base of the hypothetical plant in the figure below. "Alternate" leaves are arranged in the manner of the leaves labeled "clasping" and "decurrent" in the same drawing.

Finally, leaves are distinctive in the way they are attached to the stem. The drawing shows six common possibilities, labeled with their respective terms. Note especially that "sessile" and "petioled" are opposed terms (sessile leaves have no petioles); and that "perfoliate" leaves are pierced by the plant stem (an example is the herb boneset).

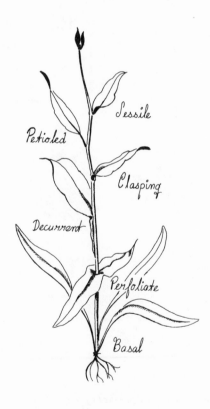

Leaf attachments

FLOWERS

Flowers, the parts of the plant that blossom and produce seeds, are classified by "inflorescence," or the way flowers are arranged on the plant stem. Flowers may be "terminal" (growing at the end of the stem or branch), or "axillary" (growing at the axil of the leaf and the stem).

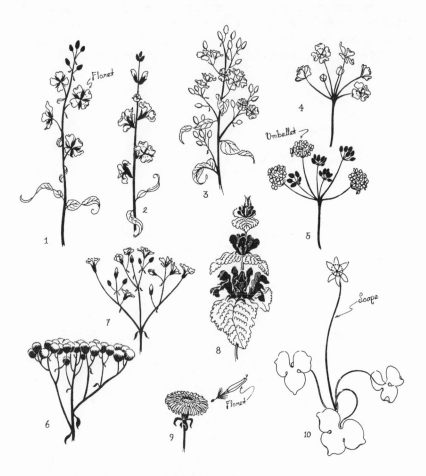

Types of inflorescence: (1) raceme; (2) spike; (3) panicle; (4) umbel; (5) compound umbel; (6) corymb; (7) cyme; (8) whorled in axil; (9) head; (10) flower on scape.

"Sessile" flowers, like sessile leaves (see above) have no stem or stalk but grow directly from the main stem or branch.

The flowers of most herbs do not grow as single blooms, but are arranged in clusters. There are many different arrangements of the small flowers ("florets") that make up flower clusters. Ten common arrangements are seen in the drawing on page 20.

FLOWER ANATOMY

The construction of flowers varies in different plant families, but in most cases flowers consist of an outer protective envelope and an inner chamber containing the seed-making parts.

The drawing shows the major flower parts. The "calyx" consists of the outer envelope of the flower's leaves ("sepals"); "corolla" is the term for the inner leaves ("petals")—often colored and showy. In the interior of the flower the "stamens" are the flower's pollen-producers (the pollen is usually borne on the head of the stamen, the "anther"). Pollen from the stamens arrives on the "pistil" at the "stigma," ultimately fertilizing the ovary within, which becomes the seed-bearing body of the plant. Most plants' flowers have stamens and pistils both, but in some plant species stamens and pistils grow separately.

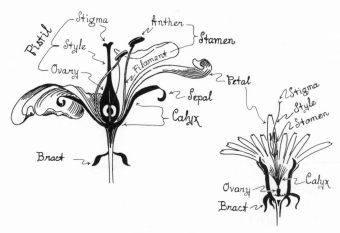

Flower parts

21

III

Where to Get Herbs

You can keep "harmless and useful herbs" in your closet in three different ways, depending on your location and life-style. But first let us describe an herb.

What is an herb? The botanical definition is a plant whose part above ground does not become woody, that dies down every year, and is valued for its medicinal properties, flavor, and scent. A spice, on the other hand, is defined as a pungent or aromatic plant used as a seasoning or preservative.

For the purposes of this book I use the standard definition of an herb as a plant, woody or otherwise, that may or may not die down every year and is used for food and medicine, drink, flavoring, preservative, or scent. A somewhat more inclusive definition which allows us to include as herbs such medicinally valuable woody plants as myrrh, wintergreen, sage, and even the eucalyptus tree.

One way to enjoy herbs is to plant an herb garden. Herbs grow happily in ordinary soil. They have only two requirements: sunshine and good drainage. They are not subject to insect pests; many of them are insect deterrents. Wormwood, tansy, garlic, onions, chives, sage, pennyroyal, nasturtiums, and marigolds are noteworthy protectors of vegetables, roses, and fruit trees.

More than half of your basic herb garden will be perennial. Many of your herbs will seed themselves, and others will develop new plants from their roots each year, enough for you to share your bounty with friends and neighbors. (See Appendix IV for a source of high-quality herb seeds and plants.)

If you enjoy walks in the country, collecting wild herbs will be a pleasant excursion across fields and meadows, through shady woods, and along fern-banked brooks. Exercise, fresh air, and a purposeful interest are all part of this free vacation package, available to everyone. If you are a city dweller, a car or bus will take you to a good area for collecting. If you live in the country or a small town, you need only walk out of your house.

DO NOT collect plants along highways where carbon monoxide has contaminated roadside herbs. DO NOT collect from under cross-country electric power lines or railroad tracks where defoliants have been used. Dirt roads, abandoned fields, and the edges of wooded areas are good places to start. Take with you a basket and larger paper or plastic bags, scissors, a knife, a trowel, a notebook, and a pencil.

For purposes of plant identification it is helpful to makes notes of where you gathered the herb. Write down the type of soil—dry, moist, sandy, gravelly, the proximity to water, sun, or shade, and the plants growing near it. The date of collection will be helpful too if you plan to go back next year. NEVER take all of any variety. If you do, the plants cannot seed themselves or spread from the roots.

The "whole herb," or everything that grows above the ground, is the useful part of some plants. The root, or that part which grows underground, is the valuable part of others.

When the bark is the useful part, never girdle the tree by taking a strip from around the trunk. Take a small perpendicular strip from one side, or from a branch.

If you want to use the magic of herbs but cannot plant or gather them, you can order the dried herbs you need from the list of reliable sources listed in the appendix.

You may want to know a little bit about the structure of the herbs

23

you grow, collect, or use. If you are faced with the need to identify an unfamiliar plant, the terminology of botany is necessary in order to understand the descriptions in the botanical texts you use for reference. The preceding chapter introduces the technical terms used to describe roots, stems, branches, leaves, and flower arrangement on the stem. You should consult plant-identification manuals if you need more detail.

IV

What Shall We Do with These Herbs?

In herbal medicine three parts of the plant are used: the root, and the underground stem or "rhizome" (those parts below the ground); what is called "the whole herb," referring to stem, leaf, and flower (those parts above the ground); and the bark.

The root should be collected in early spring, before the above-ground part has started to appear, or late in autumn when the foliage has died down. In these two seasons the important essence of the herb is in the root where, during the winter, it stores energy for near year's foliage.

The whole herb should be gathered in summer just as the plant is beginning to bloom, when it is at its peak of perfection, and when the essential essence is in foliage and blossom.

The bark should be collected in the spring when the sap is moving up from the roots to bring nourishment to the leaves.

The most common and most often used method of preparing an herb for medicinal use is called an *infusion*. This is the same method that we use in making a cup of tea. We pour two cups boiling water on one ounce of the dried herb, the equivalent of one tablespoonful, or on one loose handful of the fresh herb. Always use a ceramic, glass, or enamel container when making any herbal medicine; never use metal, particularly aluminum. Always allow the infusion to steep for ten minutes to be sure the active ingredients have been extracted. In an infusion it is usually the vitamins and volatile ingredients that are being extracted. After ten minutes pour the infusion, and, if you like, add a little pure honey to taste. It is usually not necessary to strain an herbal infusion because the leaves settle down to the bottom after ten minutes of steeping. This infusion is often referred to in herbals as a "standard brew." The correct dose is a small cupful three or four times a day. Herbs that are classified as "alteratives" are prepared in this way and are taken every day for long periods of time.

A second method of preparing herbal medicine is called a *decoction*. This is used when the plant material you want to extract is a bitter principle or mineral salt. In this method the herb, and it can be the whole herb, the root or seeds, or the bark of a woody plant is soaked in cold water for several hours, then brought to a boil and allowed to simmer for thirty minutes. The correct proportion is about one ounce of dried plant material to two cups of water. Sometimes, in the case of burdock root, for example, the dried root may be soaked in cold water overnight and the decoction made the next morning. Because a decoction is stronger than an infusion, the dose is usually one-half cup before meals. Decoctions are usually taken cool rather than hot, but if faster action is required, the first cup may be taken hot and the rest cold. Honey may be used as a sweetener.

Infusions and decoctions, both unsweetened, may be used for external application. If the infusion is used full strength and applied locally, you may dip a cloth in the liquid and wring out the excess moisture; this is call a *fomentation*. A fomentation is useful in treating a skin irritation, a headache, or an insect bite.

If a decoction is diluted in a gallon of water, this is called an *embrocation*. Embrocations are used hot and are useful for soaking a sprained ankle, foot, wrist, or finger.

A *tincture* is another method of preparation. Add one pint of pure grain alcohol or brandy to two ounces of dry (or a large handful of) fresh herbs in a glass jar. Cap the jar tightly and turn upside down. Shake the jar once or twice a day for one week. Strain and replace the liquid in the jar. This tincture will keep for six months. The dose is one tablespoonful to a wineglass of water, once or twice a day.

Honey is also a preservative, and fresh or dried herbs can be preserved in it for a month or two. This method is particularly good in preparing cough syrups. Make a concentrated infusion, eight ounces of the herb to twelve ounces of water. This is called a *standard brew concentrate*. Infuse fifteen or twenty minutes, strain and add an equal amount of honey. Horehound and coltsfoot, together or separately, make a good cough syrup used in this way. The dose is two teaspoons in one-half glass of warm water, taken three or four times a day.

Juniper berries made into a standard brew and added to herbal medicine will improve the flavor if the herb is bitter as are wormwood and boneset. Wine can also be added for flavor and will preserve the medicine for several months.

A *poultice* is a method of preparing herbs for external use. Herbs chopped fresh or dried are moistened with apple-cider vinegar and mixed with whole-wheat flour or cooked barley, the vehicle for holding it together. The proportion is one part herb to three parts vehicle. Spread the mixture on a cloth and fold the ends and sides over. The cloth should be moist and hot. Oil the skin before applying the hot poultice. A piece of plastic over it will retain the heat, or a hot pad can be used over it.

Still another type of external preparation for herbal treatment is a *salve* (for specific directions see page 188). Fresh or dried herbs are covered with water, brought to a boil, then simmered for thirty minutes. Strain and add an equal amount of olive or safflower oil. Simmer until the water has evaporated in steam, and only the oil is left. Add enough beeswax to give the mixture salve consistency and pour while hot into glass or plastic jars with tight covers. Salves will last up to a year or more.

Small cloth bags filled with such herbs as chamomile, lavender, southernwood, lemon balm, agrimony, thyme, and raspberry leaves can be put in a hot bath to relax body tensions. The fragrance will also soothe mental stress.

Since all of the preparations will be kept for some time, be sure to attach labels that will not come off and note the date of bottling as well as the ingredients.

V

Herbalists Mentioned
in Part II

Important herbalists of the past, whose works are referred to again and
again in Part II, are listed below and briefly identified.

Chapter XI, The History of Herbs, will give a more detailed account
of these herbalists and their place in the growth of herbalism. When you
read quotes from their herbals in the text, you will notice their close
observation and appreciation of plants. Many of their conclusions about
the remedial effects of herbs have been proved, by modern laboratory
tests, to have been correct.

Hippocrates, called the Father of Medicine. Greek, circa 460–circa 370 B.C.
Translations of his work are in the Loeb Classical Library.

Theophrastus, Greek, 370–287 B.C., wrote *Enquiry Into Plants.*

Pliny, Caius Plinius Secondus, A.D. 23–79, Roman naturalist, author of thirty-seven books of which only one, his *Natural History,* remains.

Dioscorides, Pedanius, of Anazarbus, author of *De Materia medica.* First century A.D., Greek physician attached to the Roman armies.

John Gerard, English, author of *The Herball, or Generall Historie of Plantes,* 1597, 1633, 1636.

Nicholas Culpepper, English, author of the *Complete Herbal,* 1652.

Thomas Greene, English, *The Universal Herbal,* 1816.

Two publications are mentioned frequently in Part II. *The United States Pharmacopeia* is published at Bethesda, Maryland. The first edition appeared December 15, 1820, in both Latin and English. Two hundred and seventeen drugs were listed. At present, the Pharmacopeia is revised every five years. A minimum of one-third of the members of the Board of Trustees and of the Committee of Revision represent the medical profession, the remainder are pharmacists.

The National Formulary is published by the American Pharmaceutical Association, Washington, D.C. It was first published in 1888, thirty-six years after the American Pharmaceutical Association was organized in 1852.

A perusal of the *United States Pharmacopeia* and the *National Formulary* from their first publication to the present time is a short course in the history of medicine and pharmacology in the United States. They contain standards of purity, a compilation of formulae, and a list of herbs used in the various formulae.

PART II

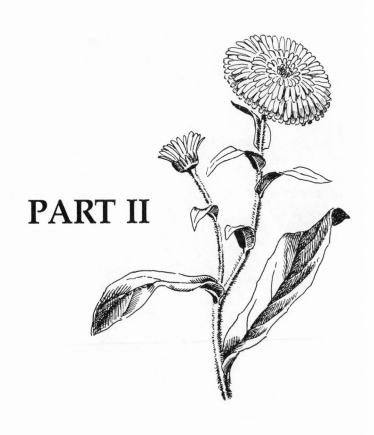

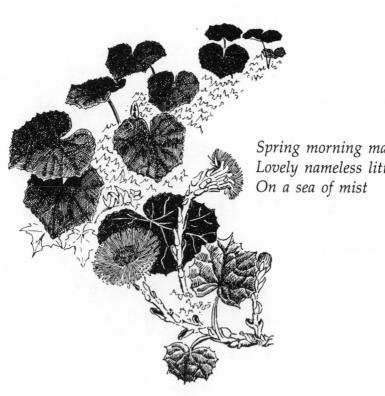

Spring morning marvel. . . .
Lovely nameless little hill
On a sea of mist

BASHO

VI

Salute to Spring

Before we salute spring, perhaps our first homage should be to Noah Webster, who, besides letting us know that spring is "a time of growth between winter and summer," tells us that "spring stresses sudden and surprising emergence especially after a period of concealed existence."

That it does, Mr. Webster. Those crisp, wavy dandelion leaves responding to the first full day of April sunshine when the garden is still a hieroglyph of brown earth, showing in squiggles through thin snow, proves to us that "sudden and surprising emergence" is the very essence of spring. An awakening and a gladness pervades our hearts and fills our lungs with deep breaths of celebration.

A practical person will now don boots and jacket and go forth to cut this welcome answer to "what's for dinner?" There will be enough tender young dandelion leaves for a large, family-sized salad. A dressing that is simple and delicious is olive oil and lemon juice, sea salt and fresh-ground pepper, a sprinkle of fresh tarragon or one-quarter teaspoon of the dried herb, the juice pressed from one clove of garlic, and a few thin slices of onion as topping.

The crowns, those round, green knobs in the center of the young leaves, which in a few weeks will rise on a long stem to support a disc of bright yellow florets, can be steamed for ten minutes and served with butter. A plate of puffy whole-wheat biscuits is the perfect accompaniment to this backyard banquet.

Sift one cup of whole-wheat flour, one cup of unbleached white flour with one teaspoon each of sea salt, baking powder, and baking soda. Mix with one-quarter cup safflower oil, and three-quarters of a cup of yogurt, plus two tablespoons of milk. Bake until golden brown in an oven preheated to 400 degrees.

This meal, health packed as it is, represents just the tip of the iceberg when we consider the other uses of the ubiquitous dandelion. When the leaves become larger (and the days longer), gather a basketful, wash, and steam them like spinach leaves. When they are barely tender, chop and serve them with butter and a dribble of apple-cider vinegar or cream, and combine with finely chopped walnuts.

The taproot of dandelion dug and dried last autumn is ready to be used as a medicinal tea if needed for hepatitis or other liver complaints. It may also be roasted and used as a coffee substitute. Frankly, I do not recommend the latter. I drink coffee infrequently, in moderate amounts, but when I do, health faddists to the contrary, I like good Colombian coffee, dark-roasted and dripped, as my French grandmother described it, "Black as night, sweet as love, and strong as the devil."

If I could choose only one wild plant for my garden, it would be milkweed, *Asclepias syriaca*—a plant for all seasons, a source of food, fiber, medicine, and esthetic pleasure, truly a vegetable survival kit.

Weeks before our garden asparagus is ready to eat, young milkweed sprouts, when they are about six inches tall, can be cut, steamed, and eaten with basil butter or any herb butter you fancy—parsley, marjoram, and chives are all good. In another week the greens will be ready to prepare as spinach.

When the milkweed buds begin to show pink, before they open into the tiny red-violet flowers that make up the corymb (flowering head), they can be steamed and served like broccoli. For a special treat, they can be made into tempura. Make a thin batter of one cup of whole-wheat pastry flour, one teaspoon arrowroot, one egg yolk, one-half teaspoon rice vinegar, and one cup water. Combine the dry ingredients and add the liquids until the batter is the right consistency, stirring lightly. Heat two cups safflower oil in an iron skillet, dip bite-sized flower heads into the batter, and fry quickly to a golden brown. Drain at once on brown paper and serve hot with or without a dip.

A dip can be made of one cup of vegetable soup stock, two table-spoons tamari or soy sauce, one tablespoon honey, fresh grated horse-radish to taste, and wild ginger root, and one tablespoon sherry. The sauce is thickened slightly with one tablespoon of arrowroot.

When the fragrant milkweed flowers have been enjoyed for several weeks in the garden where they are host to the annual pilgrimage of *Danaus plexippus*, the beautiful Monarch butterfly, milkweed has not exhausted its contribution to our health and happiness. Watch now for pale green seed pods to form. When these are one and one-half inches long, cut, wash, steam, and serve like okra. They may also be frozen and saved for winter use as a vegetable or as the perfect ingredient for a Creole gumbo, a thick seafood soup served with rice.

There is more to come. When the seed pods mature and open to reveal their white, silky threads, gather them and use the strands as an accent in wall hangings, macrame, or stitchery. The long-stapled fila-ments make a soft stuffing for small pillows, a use that our colonial forebears well knew.

Early in May, a few bright green leaf tips, rolled like a thin cigar, suddenly emerge through dark, moist earth. Comfrey, the most useful, decorative, and well-loved herb in the garden has again surrounded itself with another generation of plants that will grow up to be the image of their long-leafed, bushy mother.

Like the Victorian gardener who felt "a great pleasure in watching the ways in which different plants come through the ground,"[1] pause and enjoy these strong peaks slightly turned in at the edges, messengers of increase and renewal. Then, trowel in hand, make holes three feet apart in rich composted soil. Insert a new young plant in each hole, tucking the earth firmly around the root. Full sun, moisture, and good drainage will do the rest. In July the young plants will be as large as their mother.

In a few weeks leaves from the mother comfrey plant will be ready

[1] Henry N. Ellecombe, "A Gloucestershire Garden," a British volume on horticulture from the late nineteenth century.

to cut for salad. From this time on, throughout the spring and summer, comfrey leaves, accompanied by violet and raspberry leaves, a spring of mint, and a tablespoon of chopped orange peel, can be put in a blender filled with unsweetened pineapple juice. Liquefy this mixture for a minute or two, then pour the vitamin-filled drink over ice cubes in a tall glass and wait smugly for the inevitable delighted comments of your guests.

Another healthy and appetizing addition to the salad bowl is the stinging nettle. Early in spring when the leaves are young and tender, put on a pair of garden gloves and advance determinedly on the nearest plant, grasp it firmly, and put it in your gathering basket. If you have timed your capture correctly, the nettle will not be prickly. If you have waited a bit too long to find your nettle, all is not lost—cook it as a green. Heat disposes of the prickles.

To make a cup of nettle tea (good to stimulate the digestive juices or increase the flow of milk in nursing mothers) steep a small handful of fresh (or two teaspoons of dried) leaves in one and one-half cups of water for ten minutes. Sweeten with natural, uncooked honey.

One day in early spring, when you are removing winter mulch and tidying up the garden, you will dig the Jerusalem artichokes left in the ground last autumn. Crisp and firm after six months in nature's deep freeze, these are delicious when scrubbed, sliced very thin, and added to a salad. They have the texture of water chestnuts and more flavor. They are, like the water chestnut, a fine addition to Chinese stir-fried vegetables cooked in a wok. Add them last, so they will retain their crispness. They may also be steamed whole and served with parsley butter.

When the much-cut, yellow-green leaves of lovage are about one foot high, pointed red shoots will be seen pushing through the ground around them. Each of these shoots will make a new plant if it is dug deeply enough so that a section of root comes out with it. The young leaves of this hardy perennial that tastes like celery are a good addition to a spring salad or soup.

Salad burnet seeds itself. However, if enough young plants are not visible by the end of May, the older plants may be divided to increase your supply. The small, round, scalloped leaves have a cool cucumber taste in salad.

Sweet cicely, for all its delicate fern-like leaves and lacy white flowers, is a hardy perennial which also self-sows. Spring is the time to transplant the seedlings if they are not where you want them. The leaves of sweet cicely smell and taste like anise and are a pleasant addition to a green salad or a cole slaw. The seeds, enclosed in hard black shells, pointed at the ends, take forever to come up if you plant them. It is better to let nature do the work and then make the executive decision as to where the plants shall be.

Three herbs essential to the condiment as well as the medicine shelf must be treated as annuals in the northeast part of the United States. They are basil, marjoram, and anise. These should be started indoors, in March.

Soak peat pots in water for a few minutes, then fill them with a sterilized potting soil which has bits of pearlite in it to absorb moisture and prevent the soil from caking. Sprinkle seeds on top, cover lightly with the soil mixture, and keep the pots in a sunny window or under a grow-light. Keep them moist until the first green shows, then water very sparingly with a diluted solution of seaweed concentrate—one tablespoon to one gallon of water, used alternately with room-temperature water. This same solution may be used to water the young plants when they are transplanted into the garden; this prevents transplant shock. One gallon plastic cider jugs can be saved, and four or five kept filled with the seaweed solution, ready to use.

Some varieties of basil should be started indoors, including the common or garden variety (*Ocimum basilicum*), and the purple-leaved dark opal. In June seeds can be started in the garden for a continuous supply during the summer.

One of my favorite recipes for using basil combines it with another herb high on the list of preventive foods—garlic. To make basil pesto: Pound one and one-half cups of fresh basil and two cloves of garlic in a mortar or wooden bowl. Add three-quarters of a cup of finely grated Parmesan and one-quarter cup Romano cheese; mix to form a thick puree. When the mixture is thick and smooth, add gradually, stirring constantly, about three-quarters of a cup of olive oil. Pine nuts may be added, but pesto is excellent without them. Continue stirring until the mixture has the consistency of creamed butter. Use this as a spaghetti sauce, or on baked potatoes, noodles, or cauliflower.

One of the added pleasures of this sauce is that it can be made in advance of dinner and kept in the refrigerator until needed.

Dill, summer savory, and parsley seeds should be started outdoors as soon as the garden is ready for planting. Parsley is a biennial, which usually seeds itself in the garden. But no one wants to take a chance on having a parsley shortage. Parsley is much too valuable for food and medicine. Plant two new seed packages each year, one of the moss curled variety and one flat-leaf or Italian type. None of these herbs transplant well, so start the seeds in the garden where they are to remain. A small kitchen garden at your back door is useful, attractive, and fragrant: tall dill and summer savory in the back row, the basils, anise, and marjoram next, coriander at one end and orange mint at the other, and a double border in front of thyme and parsley.

About every fourth year you should start some new sage plants, planting the seeds in the garden where they are to stay. Sage is a hardy perennial, but the plants get woody after four or five years and should be replaced or reinforced with new ones.

A few wild herbs that you may want to have readily available in your garden can be transplanted successfully in early spring. They are: wild ginger, whose root may be used for grating in cookies, Chinese dishes, and tea; blue vervain, which is an old favorite for relieving tension; fireweed, an antispasmodic for the relief of hiccups and spasmodic coughs; and jewel weed, which is a specific for poison ivy. Consult the sections of this chapter that tell where to find these herbs and the types of soil they thrive in, then go forth armed with a pointed shovel, some large restaurant-size tin cans, and a few plastic bags. Remove both top and bottom from the cans. Loosen the soil around the plant and press the can into the soil. With the spade, dig deeply under the plant, being careful not to injure the root. The can will keep the soil pressed firmly around it. Open the large plastic bag, reach under the can with your hands, raise it and lower quickly into the plastic bag.

When you arrive home with your booty, dig a large, deep hole, fill it with water, remove the plastic bag, and gently lower the can into the hole. Pull it upwards to remove, and tamp the earth around the roots. Water heavily for three days, then only when needed.

Caution: Never take more than one plant from any one location and be sure to check the list of protected plants in your state to be sure the plants you want are not on it. If they are, you can order from a wildflower nursery (see Appendix IV). Never use manure or any fertilizer other than compost or wood humus when you transplant wild herbs.

Select a spot in your garden which corresponds closely to the natural habitat of the plant. Check the amount of sun, which direction the plant was facing (north, east, south, west), and whether the soil was rich or poor, dry or moist.

If you consult an old farmer, he will tell you to plant root crops in the dark of the moon and above-ground vegetables during the rising moon. True, but ancient wisdom has even more to offer us for guidance. It was believed that during the twenty-eight days when the moon increases from a crescent to a full moon and decreases again, it passes through the twelve signs of the zodiac. Some of these signs—Cancer, Scorpio, Pisces: the water signs—were considered fruitful signs, and, when the moon was under their influence, it was the best time to plant seeds or transplant. Aries, Gemini, Leo, Virgo, Sagittarius, and Aquarius were considered barren signs, while Libra was put in a special category, a sign under whose influence root crops could be planted safely.

ANISE

ANISE
                        Pimpinella anisum L.
                        UMBELLIFERAE

Anise has been used medicinally for at least thirty-five hundred years. A native of Egypt, it was mentioned in the Ebers Papyrus and was used in early Greek medicine.

In the United States, anise is an annual which grows up to fifteen or eighteen inches with bright green leaves, bipinnate and feathery. Seeds may be sown in the garden as soon as the soil is warm, in a spot where the plant will get direct sun most of the day.

Anise contains choline, sugar, and mucilage. Its essential oil contains up to 90 percent anethol, which gives it the typical anise fragrance and flavor. It is carminative, antiseptic, a stimulant, and a tonic.

The roots (standard decoction) reduce fever. The leaves may be cut up in salads or used as an edible garnish for lamb and pork. The seeds, the part most frequently used, are tonic and stomachic, valuable for flatulence or infant colic. They have been a popular remedy in the United States for two centuries, and we find anise listed in Jefferson's *The Family Doctor* (1869) as being recommended for the same conditions we use it for today.

Those who have not yet used anise medicinally are familiar with the seeds in cakes, cookies, and rye bread.

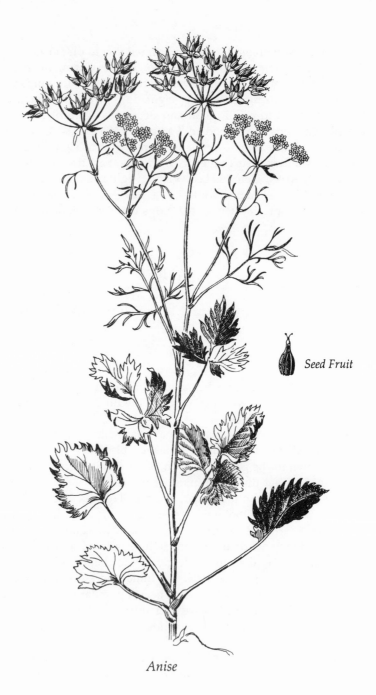

Seed Fruit

Anise

The oil is used in dentifrices as a flavor and disinfectant. Here are some suggestions for using the seeds with other herbs for healthy and delicious teas (standard brew):

Comfrey, thyme, lemon balm, and anise in equal parts
Sage, salad burnet, chickweed, and anise in equal parts
Two parts each anise and chamomile
One part each hyssop and yarrow

BASIL

SWEET BASIL	*Ocimum basilicum L.*
DWARF BASIL	*O. basilicum 'Minimum'*
DARK OPAL	*O. basilicum 'Purpurascens'*
	LABIATAE

This strong aromatic herb is, quite appropriately, under the influence of Mars, the first planet outside the earth's orbit, associated with high energy. A truly royal herb, its name is derived from the Greek word for king, basileus. In India, a species of basil (*Tulosi*, or *B. sanctum*) is sacred to Krishna and Vishnu. Planted on graves, it is every good Hindu's visa to paradise.

In Italy, the fragrant basil is given to a loved one as a pledge of fidelity, and in country districts young men wear a sprig of basil behind an ear when they go courting. The girl may respond by saying, "Baccio, carissimo," or "Kiss me, dearest." Baccio is also the common name for basil.

Ocimum basilicum came into literature with Boccaccio's famous tale from the *Decameron*, "Isabella, or the Pot of Basil." Keats's poem of the same name was written five hundred years later. A letter dated April 27, 1818, tells us that he finished the first few stanzas of "Isabella, or the Pot of Basil" but that he left them in his folio Shakespeare when he want to Teignmouth, and asked that they be sent to him. In the poem, Isabella, whose lover had been murdered by her cruel brothers, found his remains and buried them under a pot of basil "which her tears kept ever wet."

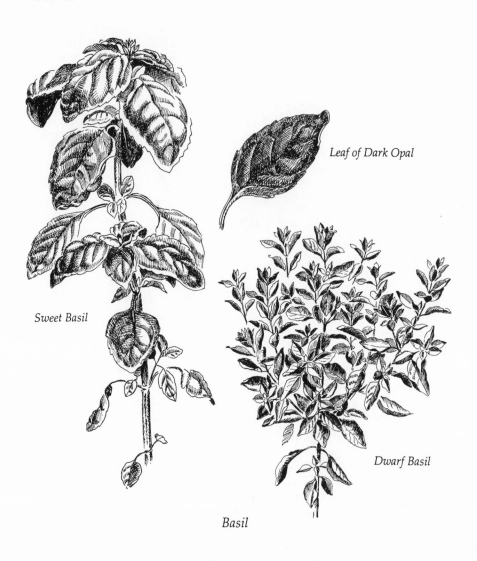

Leaf of Dark Opal

Sweet Basil

Dwarf Basil

Basil

Basil has always been a popular herb in Greece, where St. Basil's birthday on January first is celebrated. Whether there is any connection is doubtful. However, Basil the Great was born in 327 in Caesarea of Cappadocia, a part of east Asia where basil certainly thrived. The plant's geographic history traces it from India, east to Greece and Italy, and across Europe to England. From there it crossed the Atlantic to the

British colonies in America. John Winthrop, the indefatigable gardener, ordered "one ounce Bassill seeds at three pence."

Basil is a hardy annual, which can be sowed direct in the garden as soon as the soil is warm. Three varieties should find a place in every garden. The sweet or bush basil, *Ocimum basilicum*, is the one most used as a condiment. Dwarf basil makes compact little plants for a border. Just to be sure they leaf out and become bushy, pinch off the tops of the young plants. Dark opal has beautiful red-violet leaves and bluish-purple flowers and has the same fragrance as the green basils. The other basils have white flowers.

All the basils are tonic, stimulant, nervine, carminative, and disinfectant. They are used by herbalists to improve appetite, allay fatigue, and cure enteritis and intestinal catarrh.

A basil tea, standard brew, is a stimulating and refreshing drink after a hard day in the garden or at the office.

CATNIP

CATNIP   *Nepeta cataria L.*
                                                  LABIATAE

Catnip, like other mints, is under the guidance of the planet Venus, known to us as the bright star of morning and evening sky. Comfort and ease are characteristics of Venus, and catnip embodies these.

An infusion of catnip gives comfort to infants and the aging. Two to three teaspoonfuls will relieve colic and restlessness in babies; several tablespoonfuls can dispose of gastric pains and flatulence in adults.

The whole herb is carminative, diaphoretic, antispasmodic, tonic, emmenagogue, and mildly nervine.

It relieves colds and fevers by inducing perspiration and helps the body to regain its balance by its calming effect, allowing the patient to get much-needed sleep.

The infusion, taken internally, is good for both reducing the pain of menstrual cramps and curing headache. As a fomentation, it is useful in reducing swelling caused by sprains or insect bites.

43

Catnip is a hardy perennial, which grows to three feet tall in the garden; its many-branched, square stem has opposite gray-green leaves, small, heart-shaped, and deeply serrated. Lavender flowers on graceful spikes bloom in July and August in northern New England. The fresh leaves do not exude the typical catnip flavor unless they are bruised or dried. My cat ignores the growing plant, but is delighted with catnip balls made out of the dried leaves. A wild variety which is taller and has larger leaves and white flowers grows in Vermont.

Catnip tea will prevent a cold if you drink a cup of the warm infusion, sweetened with honey, when you notice the slightest symptom. It counteracts fatigue and improves circulation. Do not go out in the cold after drinking it; get in bed and cover up, preferably with an old-fashioned down quilt. Why a down quilt? Because it is very warm and very light. When treating a cold, you should be as warm and as comfortable as

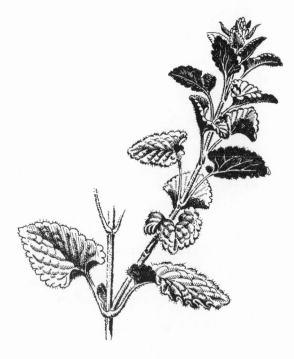

Catnip

possible. Heavy blankets weigh down on your body and have a depressing effect. I will anticipate the question, what about an electric blanket? An electric blanket satisfies the requirements, being light and warm. If your electricity rate is not as exorbitant as mine, use one by all means.

The first dry, sunny day after the lavender flowers have opened, cut catnip stalks for drying. Both wild and cultivated varieties have the same properties, and both are suitable for preventive and curative uses.

A healthy winter tea for prevention and enjoyment is made by infusing standard brew: equal quantities of catnip, comfrey, and red clover with half the amount of sage.

CHAMOMILE

ROMAN CHAMOMILE   *Chamaemelum nobile* (L.) Ait.
                    (Anthemis nobilis L.)
GERMAN CHAMOMILE   *Matricaria recutita* L.
                    (M. chamomilla L.proparte,
                    Chamomilla recutita [L.]
                    Rauschert)

                                    COMPOSITAE

This well-known little plant is under the protection of the sun, and it thrives gratefully in a location where it gets direct sunshine. It is low-growing, seldom more than ten inches in height. The jointed, fibrous root sends up a many-branched, tender stem. The leaves are finely cut and minute daisy-like flowers appear singly on erect stalks, the florets white, the centers yellow. German chamomile is an annual; Roman chamomile is a perennial.

Chamomile plants, placed around the garden in small groups, will insure the health of other plants. An ailing herb or vegetable can be restored to health by setting a chamomile plant next to it.

It is the flower heads that are used medicinally. The active principles are primarily in the volatile oil.

Chamomile is tonic, stomachic, anodyne, and antispasmodic. The tea, made as a standard brew, is soothing, sedative, and completely harmless. One teaspoonful to one cup of liquid may be given to babies as a remedy for colic. It is also good for adults in cases of upset stomach, alone or in combination with lemon balm (melissa), peppermint, anise, fennel, or caraway.

That chamomile was highly thought of in sixteenth-century England we know from Gerard's praise of it. "A decoction made of Camomile, and drank, takes away all pains and stitches in the side. . . . The bathing with a decoction of Camomile takes away weariness, loses pains, to what part of the body soever they be applied. It comforts the sinews that are over-strained, mollifies all swellings: It moderately comforts all parts that have need of warmth, digests and dissolves whatsoever has need thereof, by a wonderful speedy property. It eases all pains of the cholic and stone, and all pains and torments of the belly and gently provokes urine."

Gerard also tells us that, "This is Nechessa, an Egyptian's medicine."

A bag of chamomile heads and leaves put in a hot bath will help ease pain in every part of the body and is a relief for excessive fatigue.

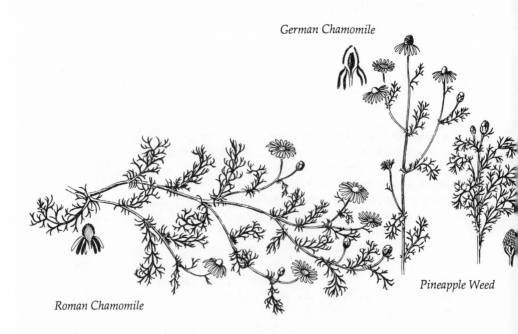

German Chamomile

Pineapple Weed

Roman Chamomile

Chamomile

Cosmetically, chamomile is an excellent rinse for blond hair, restoring its natural color and giving it a healthy sheen.

A combination of the flower heads and poppy seeds makes an effective fomentation for external use in treating swellings and neuralgia. This mixture has both antiseptic and painkilling qualities.

In New England there is a wild chamomile, known locally as "pineapple weed," botanically called *Matricaria matricarioides*, a common ground cover with little, round, yellow buttons, and rayless heads. It was naturalized in New England from the West Coast, California, and the Rocky Mountains.

German chamomile, *Matricaria recutita*, is sometimes called wild chamomile. It is taller than the Roman variety and the flower heads are somewhat larger, about three-quarters of an inch across.

All varieties of chamomiles have the same medicinal properties and can be used to treat the same problems.

CHERVIL

CHERVIL   *Anthriscus cerefolium* L.,Hoffm.

                                          UMBELLIFERAE

A low-growing annual, ten to twelve inches high, chervil is hardy in New England winters if it is planted in the fall and not allowed to go to seed. Its fernlike leaves and ribbed stems give it the appearance of an aristocratic parsley; it is often called, imprecisely but understandably, "queen of the parsleys."

Known to cooks throughout the world as a flavorful addition to sauces, salad dressings, and soups, chervil must be used fresh to produce its full flavor. Since cooking destroys both its aroma and its color, chervil is always added last to cooked foods.

Try adding a handful of finely chopped fresh chervil to a potato soup made as follows: Cook until tender a few chopped potatoes and a clove of garlic in just a little water (enough to cover the potatoes). Put through a food mill, add two cups of medium cream and salt and pepper to taste. Reheat until almost boiling, remove from the fire, and add the chopped chervil.

47

In America chervil is better known for its culinary virtue than for its medicinal quality. In France and Spain it is used by herbalists to clear the liver and kidneys, to help the passing of stones, for colic and other digestive problems, and to dissolve blood clots. For all these purposes it should be eaten raw, sprinkled on bread or cooked foods. The fresh leaves, macerated and placed directly on a painful bruise, will give relief.

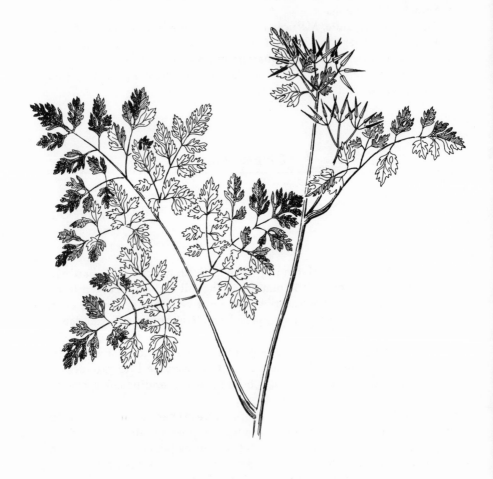

Chervil

COLTSFOOT

COLTSFOOT   *Tussilago farfara L.*
                                                     COMPOSITAE

This hardy perennial is found in Europe, the United States, and the East Indies. It grows wild in wet areas, along stream banks or pastures, on embankments, and in almost any loamy and limestone soil.

The botanical name, *Tussilago,* means "cough dispeller," and the common name "coltsfoot" refers to the shape of the round leaves. The plant contains tannin, mucilage, and a bitter amorphous glucoside. It is mucilaginous, demulcent, expectorant, tonic, astringent, and emollient.

Coltsfoot, unlike most plants, does not flower while it is in leaf. The flowers come first, in early spring, large, radial, yellow blossoms on downy-white, scaly stems. As the flowers begin to wilt, large, round, cordate-shaped leaves appear which are cottony white underneath and smooth or glabrous on the top. The flowers should be collected as soon as they are in bloom, the leaves immediately upon attaining full size. Dioscorides, Galen, Pliny, and many authorities of all ages have put their stamp of approval on the smoking of coltsfoot leaves for the cure of a cough. Cotton Mather also recommended it for "sweetening the blood."

In England a tobacco is made which allows those with respiratory problems to enjoy smoking without harm. It contains coltsfoot, buck bean, eyebright, betony, rosemary, thyme, lavender, and chamomile flowers. This will afford relief of asthma and any difficult breathing due to bronchitis, catarrh, or other respiratory cause.

An effective cough syrup can be made using honey as the base and adding strong decoctions of coltsfoot, horehound, ground ivy (prunella), comfrey, and pennyroyal. Other combinations can be made to fit treatment of the specific type of cough and the physical condition of the person to be treated.

You will notice by reading the characteristics of coltsfoot that it is both emollient and expectorant. It will soothe the tissues of the throat as well as cause phlegm to be expelled. If a patient is inclined to have indigestion, the addition of peppermint may be indicated. Read the end of Chapter I again before you prescribe or make herbal formulas.

Decoctions or infusions of coltsfoot may be applied externally to the

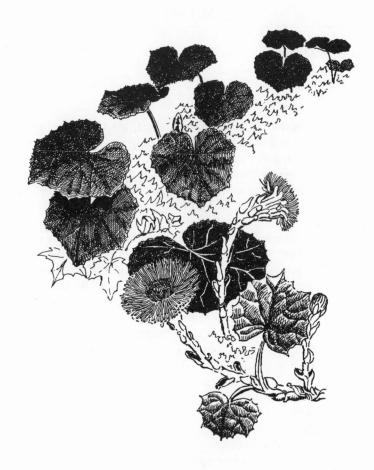

Coltsfoot

pulmonary region as either a hot compress or poultice. For a compress, soak flannel cloth in standard brew. For a poultice, make according to directions in Chapter IV.

To make coltsfoot cough drops, boil one ounce fresh leaves in one pint water until only one cupful is left. Strain, add two cups of sugar and boil until a drop forms a hard ball in cold water. Pour onto a buttered cookie sheet, score into cough drop sizes. Roll in slippery elm powder so the drops will not be sticky.

COMFREY

COMFREY   *Symphytum officinale* L.
BORAGINACEAE

Comfrey is a hardy perennial under the protection of the planet Saturn. The botanical name, *Symphytum,* is derived from the Greek word meaning "to grow together" and refers to the mucilaginous root which does just that—causes torn flesh and bones to unite.

Culpepper says of comfrey, "The root boiled in water and wine, and the decoction drank, heals inward hurts, bruises, wounds and ulcers of the lungs, and causes the phlegm that oppresses them to be easily spit forth. . . . The roots being outwardly applied cure fresh wounds or cuts immediately, being bruised and laid thereto; and is specially good for ruptures and broken bones, so powerful to consolidate and knit them together that if boiled with dissevered pieces of flesh in a pot, it will join them together again."

It is not often that we can add to the exuberant claims of this seventeenth-century astrologer–physician, but in the case of comfrey we can say that the leaves, if applied fresh to cuts will also heal them, take out the pain, stop the bleeding, and prevent bruising.

Comfrey has been used for more different curative purposes than any other plant, and more importantly, the claims made for it have held up under present-day scrutiny. Literally a one-herb pharmacy, it is emollient, astringent, alterative, expectorant, vulnerary, pectoral, healing for any kind of respiratory disease. It is also a cell proliferant (increases cell growth), and is healing for internal and external use.

Comfrey root is high in mucilage, containing even more than the marsh mallow. It also contains allantoin and a small amount of starch and tannin. The allantoin content in aqueous solution has a powerful action in strengthening epithelial formations, or protecting any injured tissues, external or internal. It build healthy cells which heal external wounds and ulcers of the stomach or duodenum.

This wonder plant contains potassium, calcium, phosphorus, iron, magnesium, and cobalt. It is rich in Vitamin B (nicotinic and pantothenic acids, and riboflavin), Vitamin B_{11} (thiamin), and B_{12} (cobalamin). Comfrey also contains Vitamins C and E.

Specific ailments that comfrey has benefited are: arthritis, asthma,

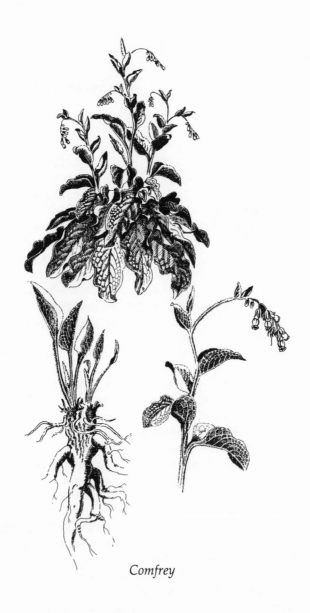

Comfrey

athletes' foot, bed sores, swollen joints, piles, sprains, cuts, open wounds, bee stings, bronchitis, and bruises.

The species of comfrey known as *S.* x *uplandicum* is the best for garden cultivation. The leaves are less coarse than the wild comfrey, it has handsome blue to purplish blossoms and grows in a lush, well-shaped mound. The original plants of prickly comfrey, *S. asperum*, were introduced into England by Henry Doubleday about 1870. They were sent to him by one of the British or Scotch successors to Joseph Bush, head gardener to Catherine the Great, who laid out and planted the gardens of St. Petersburg Palace, the present Park of Rest and Culture in Leningrad. In the latter years of the nineteenth century, growers in England were getting a yield of eighty to one hundred tons an acre from what they called "Russian comfrey," *S. x uplandicum*, to distinguish it from Henry Doubleday's original import. Investigations by the Cambridge Botanic Gardens have shown that this "Russian comfrey" was a natural hybrid between *S. asperum* and *S. officinale*, the common comfrey native to England, Europe, and Russia. It is an F hybrid like many of the new and improved vegetable varieties. As in many of the new hybrids, the tissue that fits together over the stamens and around the base of the pistil fails to open, preventing the entry of bees. Therefore, root division (one of the three types of clone propagation) is the only way to insure a plentiful supply of identical plants.

The plant grows two to three feet high. The lower leaves are large, ten to sixteen inches long, ovate, lanceolate, pointed and slightly wavy, hairy, with veins and veinlets clearly defined. The upper leaves are smaller, the stem branched, terminating in one-sided clusters of drooping, bee-shaped flowers that grow on only one side of the stem. The racemes are paired and half-moon curved. Buds nearest the main stalk of the plant open first.

In New England, comfrey blooms in July. The handsome, blue-blossomed flower stalks make a decorative background or corner plant in the garden so a few should be allowed to flower. But for use as food, animal fodder or herbal medicine, the stalks should be cut back before they flower and the large basal leaves harvested two or three times a growing year, cut to within two inches of the base of the plant. The first cutting, in New England, can usually be made at the end of June.

The root of comfrey is long and spindle shaped, fibrous and fleshy. The outside is smooth and dark colored, the inside white and juicy.

There is no waste to comfrey. Last season's wilted leaves, after a heavy frost, are dug into the ground to prepare it for this year's bed of tomatoes. Any mud-streaked lower leaves, unfit for food or drying, are used as a top dressing. Comfrey is an ideal fertilizer for tomatoes because it contains three times as much potash as it does nitrogen and far less phosphorus.

Comfrey is an excellent home treatment for flu and bronchitis. Make

53

a standard brew concentrate of two parts comfrey, one part yarrow, one part boneset, and a few juniper berries.

For diarrhea or dysentery, simmer one ounce of dried comfrey root in one pint of milk. Take a wineglassful three times a day.

For a cough make this mixture: soak two ounces of comfrey root in one quart of water, overnight. Bring to a boil and simmer thirty minutes. Strain, add six ounces of honey and two ounces glycerin and simmer again for five minutes. Cook, store in a glass jar and take one tablespoonsful three or four times a day.

To alleviate skin problems, bed sores, athletes' foot, a useful salve can be made. The directions and ingredients are given in Chapter VIII, Autumn.

In the late 1970s, comfrey got a bad press. Experimental data from Australia were said to indicate that laboratory rats which had been fed comfrey showed liver damage due to pyrrolizidine alkaloids. A careful evaluation of this material was done by John Pembery, research chemist, and published by Lawrence D. Hills as a special report to the Henry Doubleday Research Association of England. The rats whose livers were affected had been fed several times their body weight of comfrey leaves over a long time. It has been calculated that it would take "140 years of drinking four cups of comfrey tea a day for a person to run the risk of alkaloid poisoning."

The danger that this will happen to any human being seems minimal. Of course, it must always be considered that some people may be allergic to food that is quite safe for the majority (as is shown by those few who get hives from eating strawberries).

DANDELION

DANDELION   *Taraxacum officinale* L.
                                                    COMPOSITAE

Whether the dandelion is a native American or a naturalized plant is debated by authorities. Certainly it is found and eaten in most parts of the world. At least two reports from the early nineteenth century attest to its use here. Joseph Smith listed it as "aperient and deobstruent" and said that it "opens the system in general."[1] In the "Report on Medical Botany,"[2] Dr. Clapp tells us that in 1852 dandelion was used "in chronic diseases of the liver." This use has proved well justified, as the plant has been found to contain taraxacin, a hepatic stimulant; inulin; a sugar, lacvulin; choline, one of the Vitamin B complex; photosterols, which prevent the body from accumulating cholesterols; and potash, which is a diuretic.

In Peking, in the Hospital of Traditional Medicine, we were shown Chin Hung tablets and told that these were a specific for appendicitis. The formula includes *Taraxacum mongolicum,* the Chinese dandelion, and three other ingredients. The tablets have a reasonably good record. Eighty percent of the patients recover without an operation. Five percent come to the hospital too late to avoid an operation because the appendix is near to bursting. Fifteen percent have a recurrence but are cured by a second course of medication with Chin Hung.

All parts of the dandelion are used today, the roots for hepatitis, the leaves and crowns for salads and cooked greens, the flowers for making wine, and the juice to cure warts and blisters.

The Latin name for dandelion was *dens leonis* and the French name of *dent de lion* evolved in English to the present "dandelion." The reason for these names is the somewhat imaginative resemblance of the deeply-serrated leaf to a lion's tooth. The leaf of the plant varies. In some it is deeply cut, in others wavy rather than toothed. The taproot is thick, the exterior brown, the inside milky white. A hollow, smooth, red-tinged stem grows up straight from the middle of a rosette of leaves that lies flat to the ground, and bears yellow, strap-shaped florets. When these are broken off the stem exudes a milky juice. Dandelion watchers report that no less than eighty-five different insects banquet on its pollen.

In early spring when our bodies seem to cry out for fresh greens, the tender, young dandelion leaves make a welcome salad. John Burroughs, in *A Year in the Fields*, wrote, "I plucked my first dandelion on a meadow slope on the twenty-third (of May)." See Chapter VI, Salute to Spring, for directions for preparing dandelion leaves and crowns.

Both the dried leaves and the dried and powdered root are used as

---

[1] Joseph Smith, *The Dogmaticus, Or Family Physician.* Rochester, New York: Marshall and Dean, 1829.

[2] "Report on Medical Botany," Transactions of the American Medical Association, V.

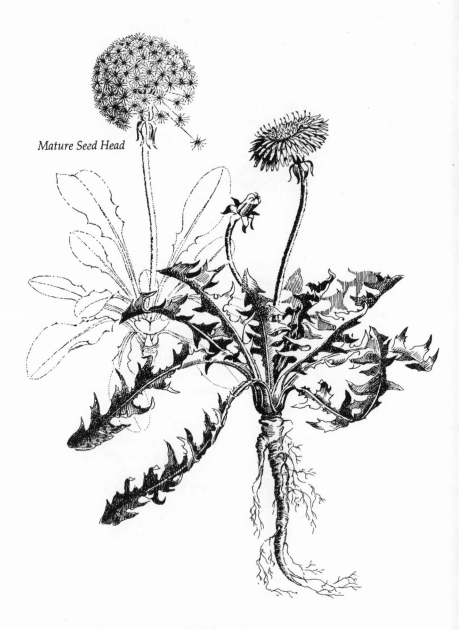

Mature Seed Head

Dandelion

tea. Prepare the leaves as an infusion and the root as a decoction. The tea is a specific for hepatitis and any malfunction of the liver.

On a dry day in summer when the sun's rays turn a field of dandelions into shining gold discs, take a bushel basket with you and walk through the field. Snip off perfect blossoms as you go, enjoying the sun, until your basket is full. The ones you cut will not be missed in the sea of color.

Colonial households enjoyed a wine made from dandelion flowers. In Chapter VII, Summer: Gourmet Gardening, I give a recipe for this wine.

Dandelions, fresh leaves or dried root, are valuable additions to a diet for diabetics. Add lettuce to the raw greens, steep juniper berries with the powdered root; both are good, as in dandelion, for reducing the sugar count.

When the first issue of the *National Formulary* came out in 1888, it listed a "compound elixir of Taraxacum" in twelve different formulas, and the listing continued until 1965. The dried root was official until 1926 in the *United States Pharmacopeia*.

If you have always thought about dandelions as weeds, perhaps you can see them now as edible tonics and digestive aids, as stimulants for both liver and lymph glands. One last hurrah for the dandelion—it is a treatment for mononucleosis.

FIREWEED

FIREWEED   *Epilobium angustifolium* L.
("WILLOWEED")

ONAGRACEAE

The perennial, willowlike leaves of fireweed grow quick and tall to cover bulldozed or burnt-over ground, its bright pink blossoms a badge of nature's rural renewal program. No soil is too thin, poor or unlikely for fireweed. In front of my house there is a steep bank where soil is not more than an inch deep above granite ledge, with outcroppings of rock. Here fireweed has taken over to give pink summer protection from dust on the road below it, and in autumn wavy, gray-bearded seed plumes remain attractive until heavy snows weigh them down.

Demulcent, astringent, tonic, and antispasmodic, fireweed has its

57

medicinal as well as aesthetic uses. The leaves and flowers, steeped in safflower oil for three days, are a soothing local application for piles.

A decoction of the whole herb may be taken for hiccups, whooping cough, or other spasmodic coughs. The dose, taken cold, is one-half cup at a time until the paroxysms pass.

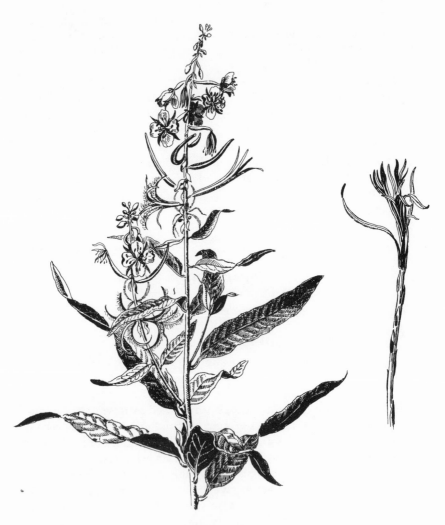

Fireweed

GINGER

WILD GINGER   *Asarum canadense* L.
ARISTOLOCHIACEAE

Wild ginger, *Asarum canadense,* is a native American plant, whose medicinal qualities were known to many Indian tribes. The Rappahannocks steeped the leaves to reduce fever in typhoid. For treatment of a fractured arm, the Ojibwa Indians used a warm poultice of wild ginger and spikenard (*Aralia racemosa*), covered by a cloth and bound with fitted cedar splints. The Hopis used a decoction of boiled root and rhizomes as an oral contraceptive. It was thought to induce temporary sterility, but no scientific findings have validated this use. This was two hundred years before "modern medicine" experimented with oral contraceptives.

Asarum canadense is aromatic, tonic, carminative, stimulant, and diaphoretic. The dried root was official in the *United States Pharmacopeia* from 1820–73, and it was listed in the *National Formulary* until 1947. According to Dr. Edward P. Claus, two antibiotic substances have been isolated from wild ginger, one of which is an active deterrent to pus-forming bacteria.

As a diaphoretic, wild ginger is recommended in cases of inflammation or obstruction of the lungs, spleen, bowels, kidneys, bladder, or uterus to equalize circulation. It can be used in a vapor bath or as an infusion. One-half ounce of the powdered root in one pint of boiling water, steeped fifteen minutes, should be taken, hot, to induce perspiration. The leaves have been classified as a powerful emetic. I have not tried this, but would not hesitate to do so if such an emetic were indicated, as the leaves are readily available, fresh in summer, dried in winter.

The large, heart-shaped leaves of the wild ginger grow on short stems and hide the small, trumpet-shaped, red-umber colored flower which rests on the ground beneath them. The plant is found in rich, damp soil and spreads rapidly in a situation congenial to it. I have transplanted it from the woods to a shady, protected slope where it has begun to increase despite competition from nearby day lilies.

I use the dried, scraped root in cooking as a substitute for the real ginger, *Zingiber officinale*, which, in our climate, can be raised only as an indoor pot plant.

One tablespoonful of grated, wild ginger root, a clove of garlic put through a press, and one-half cup of Tamari (soy sauce) used as a

59

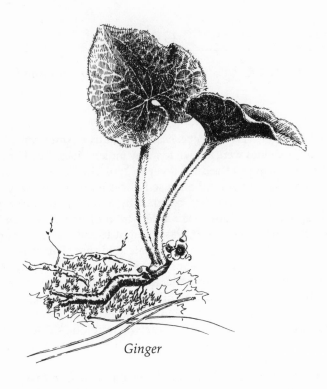

Ginger

marinade for pork chops before they are broiled makes this dish a gour-met treat. Serve with steamed yams and applesauce.

Add grated or powdered wild ginger to other herbal teas for added stimulus to circulation in the winter.

JEWEL WEED

JEWEL WEED   *Impatiens capensis* Meerb.
("BALSAM WEED," "WILD BALSAM,"
"SPOTTED TOUCH-ME-NOT")

BALSAMINACEAE

These tall annual plants with weak, pale green stems and thin-tex-tured, ovate, pointed leaves grow from one and a half to two and a half

Empty Seed Pod

Flowers and Seed Pods

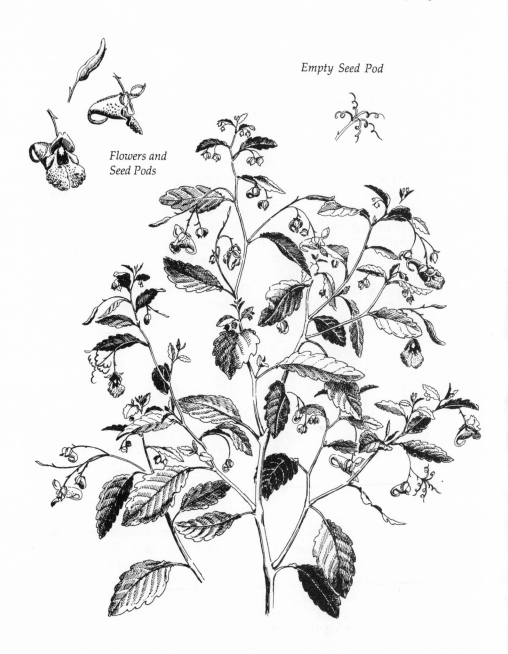

Jewel Weed

61

feet high. Their slipper-shaped orange flowers sprinkled with reddish-brown spots resemble a columbine emulating the colors of a tiger lily. It is from the seed pods, which, when ripe, explode their seeds by elastic separation and uncoiling of valves, that the plant gets its name, *Impatiens.* Goldfinch seem to know, instinctively, when the surprising rain of seeds will occur and, in my garden, are always on hand to catch them.

The fresh juice of the plant is a specific for poison ivy. The bruised leaves and stems may be applied directly to the sores caused by poison ivy or made into a poultice with slippery elm and cider vinegar.

If space in your garden permits, it is nice to allow a small bed of jewel weed to become established, an easy thing to do as the goldfinch always drop a few seeds. The plant has three things to recommend it: the beauty of its flowers, the ready availability of a remedy for poison ivy, and the assurance of an annual visit of flocks of goldfinch.

Jewel weed is native to North America, where it grows from coast to coast and north from Mexico to Canada. It is also found along some of the southern waterways of England. John Burroughs wrote in 1875, "Our beautiful jewel-weed has recently appeared along certain of the English rivers."

LOVAGE

LOVAGE   *Levisticum officinale* Koch
                                                    UMBELLIFERAE

A member of the same family as dill, angelica, and parsley, lovage is a hardy perennial under the planetary influence of the Sun, whose rays call attention to its bright chartreuse foliage in June.

The botanical name, *Levisticum,* can be translated "from Liguria," and refers to the place of origin. The Romans, who knew a good thing when they saw it, brought lovage from the Ligurian coast of Italy to Britain.

The plant grows from three to six feet tall. The green stems are hollow, and the leaves compound, much divided. The whole plant may

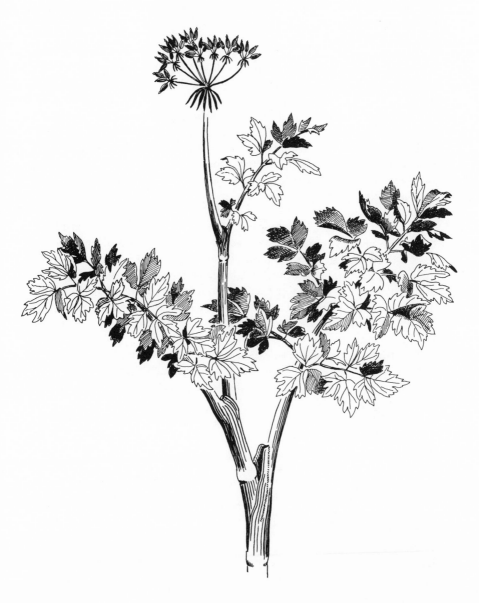

Lovage

best be described by saying that it looks, smells, and tastes more like celery than celery. In the garden it is a good background plant and is at its best before the flower stalk shoots up tall above the bright foliage. The umbels of yellow flowers are attractive but soon turn into brown, elliptical, curved seeds with winged ribs. As both leaves and seeds are valuable, they should be gathered while in their prime, leaves first, the seeds just as they begin to ripen.

Lovage came to America with the early English colonists. It may be seen, and studied, in Plymouth Plantation Gardens, where a careful restoration of a Pilgrim Village is open to the public. It was brought over for food and medicine. Celery was harder to establish in the cold Massachusetts winters, and lovage was used as a celery substitute as well as a digestive, a carminative, and a stomachic, to cure jaundice, and "to cleanse humors."

It had other virtues. Culpepper, that redoubtable astrologer–physician of Spitalfields, said, "It takes away the redness and dimness of the eyes if dropped into them; it removes spots and freckles from the face."

In the Scandinavian countries, lovage is used today as a complexion aid. Washing the face with lovage water is cleansing and refreshing, and gives tone to the skin. Combined with rue, it is efficient in the treatment of acne, used as a tea taken internally, twice a day, and as a local application.

English public houses used to serve a cordial made with lovage, tansy, and yarrow. A tea, made from the same ingredients, in the proportion of two parts lovage and yarrow and one part tansy, is excellent as a general tonic.

Lovage leaves, dried and crumbled, are a tasty addition to a winter soup or stew, giving a celery flavor when celery is expensive in the food stores. Fresh green leaves are delicious in a salad, and the hollow stems, split and cut in two-inch pieces, can be filled with cream cheese for hors d'oeuvres or as an addition to a sandwich plate. The cheese can be given a variety of flavors by the addition of curry powder, sesame, anise, chives, and/or soy sauce.

Lovage does well when started from seeds, but the mother herb is encircled each spring with eager, healthy, young plants, which can be transplanted to rich soil in a spot that gets at least half a day of direct sun. Young leaves should be ready to cut by the end of June or the first week in July. Chopped leaves and stalks give flavor and texture to both potato and chicken salad. Cooked in a wok, lovage blends well with other vegetables in Chinese dishes.

Lovage can be enjoyed even at the end of the gardening season. When the leaves, yellow-green in the summer, turn mustard yellow to copper brown (the tones of a Harunobi print), they are a very special part of the autumn scene, a subject to photograph before cutting back just a few inches above the ground. It is good gardening practice to heap the cut branches around the base of each plant to form a winter mulch. What a satisfying feeling it is to help nature to do things in her immemorial way.

MARJORAM

SWEET MARJORAM *Origanum majorana* L.
OREGANO *Origanum vulgare* L.
("WILD MARJORAM")

LABIATAE

Wild marjoram is stimulant, carminative, diaphoretic, mildly tonic and emmenagogic. It is a strong herb used as a rubefacient and a lini-

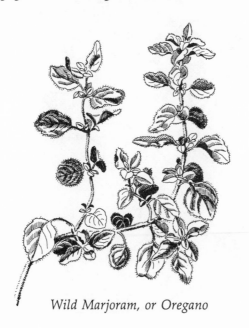

Wild Marjoram, or Oregano

65

ment. Greek medicine used wild marjoram externally in fomentations and internally as a tea for convulsions and dropsy, and as an antidote for narcotic poisons.

Today we use the warm infusion (standard brew) to relieve colic, spasms, and dyspeptic pain. These uses are not new—they appeared in most family medicine books of the nineteenth century. A warm infusion

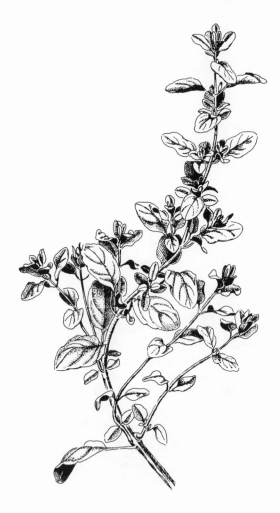

Sweet Marjoram

is given in the early stages of measles to promote perspiration and bring out the rash. A few drops of oil from the leaves can be put in the hollow of an aching tooth to relieve pain.

Wild marjoram, or what we call today oregano, is a hardy garden perennial, which grows to a bushy shrub sometimes eighteen to twenty-four inches high. The flowers have a two-lipped, light purple corolla, a five-toothed calyx and grow in corymbs, which usually bloom in July and August in New England.

Sweet marjoram is a dainty, low, shrubby plant with woody stems and delicate, oval, opposite leaves and white flowers. In Portugal, its native land, sweet marjoram is a perennial; but in cold climates it must be treated as an annual and started every spring from seed, indoors, or in a well-protected cold frame.

It is a fragrant culinary herb used in soups and stews, meat, egg, and cheese dishes, sauces, herb butter, and homemade mayonnaise.

The Spanish colonists of the western United States used marjoram in many dishes, as they did sage, and as the French colonists of the southern states used bay, thyme, and cayenne.

If potted before cold weather, sweet marjoram will live through the winter on a sunny window sill where the leaves can be snipped for flavoring. Both species may be dried, quick frozen, or salted on a tray in an oven at a temperature of 150 degrees.

MILKWEED

MILKWEED   *Asclepias syriaca* L.
                                                ASCLEPIADACEAE

Milkweed, an herbaceous plant that exudes milky juice, grows to three feet high and, in spite of its misleading descriptive name *"syriaca,"* is a native of the United States and Canada. The deep rose-colored flower heads are handsome and sweet smelling.

Milkweed is diuretic, emetic, and purgative. It is helpful in asthma and systemic catarrh to produce expectoration and relieve pain and coughing. Not surprisingly, milkweed was used by the American Indians. One tribe cured warts with the milky juice. Another used infusions

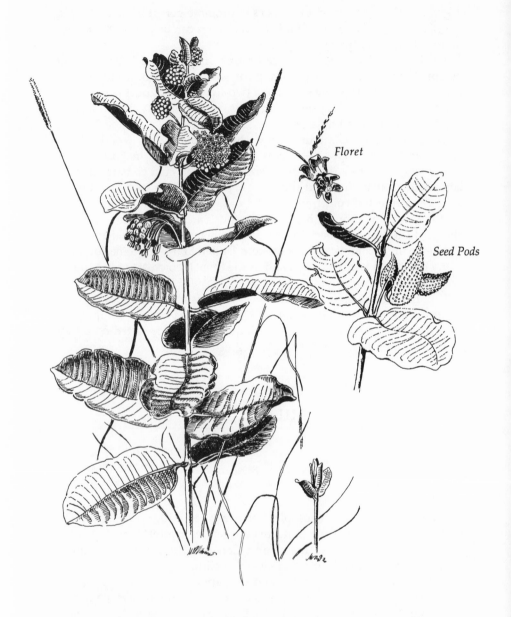

Floret

Seed Pods

Milkweed

of the root to produce temporary sterility. This was obviously successful as students of Indian culture have reported that the average Indian family was two, never more than three children.

Constituents of milkweed are asclepione (a crystalline substance), fatty matter, caoutchouc, gum, sugar, and some salts.

Pleurisy root (*Asclepias tuberosa*), also called "butterfly weed," is another of the approximately eighty *Asclepias*. A handsome plant that grows to one and one-half feet high, it is different from other plants of the species in that it is devoid of the characteristic milky juice. Deep yellow to orange flowers are born on large corymbs in September.

The root of butterfly weed contains a glucoside (asclepiadin), several resins, fatty matter, and a trace of volatile oil. It is antispasmodic, diaphoretic, expectorant, tonic, carminative, and mildly cathartic. It is recommended in diarrhea, dysentery, acute and chronic rheumatism, and eczema. Large doses should be avoided because they are emetic and purgative. Small, frequent doses of an infusion of the root will increase perspiration and ease expectoration.

The milkweeds (*Asclepias*) were named for Aesculapius, who is said to have learned his knowledge of healing from an apprenticeship to Cheiron, the centaur whose herbal and medical skills came direct from Apollo. In any case, by the eighth century B.C. Aesculapius had been made a god, and his methods of healing spread from his Temple at Epidaurus to the far borders of Asia Minor. The healing, fragrant, helpful milkweeds are a fitting tribute to his memory.

MINT

SPEARMINT	*Mentha spicata* L.
PEPPERMINT	*M.* x *piperita* L.
PENNYROYAL	*M. pulegium* L.
	LABIATAE

Spearmint, peppermint, and pennyroyal are the most important species of mints. They are all under the protection of the Moon, which traditionally also controlled human breasts and stomach. Certainly the

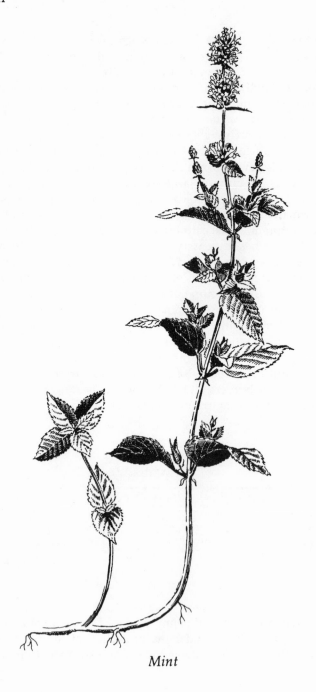

Mint

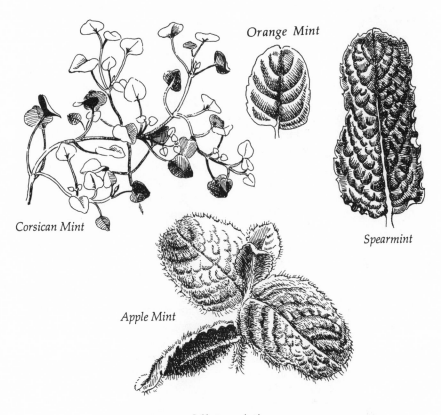

Orange Mint

Corsican Mint

Spearmint

Apple Mint

Mint varieties

mints have long been noted for their beneficent effect on the digestive system.

The family of mints has been used and valued since the beginning of written history and before. Mint, with anise and cumin, was the tithe paid by the Pharisees. It appears in every list of herbs that has come down to us—Egyptian, Greek, Roman, medieval, and American colonial.

Mint was an important "strewing herb" for which use Gerard says, "the smelle rejoiceth the heart of man." In seventeenth-century England, it was strewn in the court rooms to protect the judges from germs and stench when prisoners were brought in from the highly unsanitary gaols.

Part II

Because of its ancient and modern cultivation, all over the world mint is found as a garden escapee, growing wild in damp fields and following streams wherever man has lived. There are more different varieties than the most astute botanist can identify, as mint cross-pollinates readily.

Culpepper lists some forty ills that mint will cure. During the Renaissance it was used to whiten the teeth and it is used today as an ingredient in many toothpastes, in soap, and in skin lotions.

The mints are stimulant, carminative, antispasmodic, diuretic, and febrifuge. As preventive medicine, they should have a place in kitchens as well as in medicine chests—as tisanes or tea for daily use, in sauces, and as additions to vegetables and salads, soups, and cool fruit drinks.

A wild variety grows in Mexico, where it is called "herba boracho" (herb of drunks), and bunches of it are handed to guests at village weddings to prevent intoxication and to aid digestion.

In the United States, spearmint is best known as mint jelly, as the green sprig in a mint julep, and as the flavor in spearmint chewing gum. It has lanceolate, wrinkled, bright green leaves, which contain oil of spearmint, whose principal ingredient is carvone. It also contains phellandrene, limonene, and dihydro-carveol acetate. Other ingredients are esters of acetic, butyric, and caproic acids.

Peppermint, a red-stalked, dark green, pointed-leafed mint, contains oil of peppermint, the chief constituent of which is menthol. It also contains menthyl acetate and isovalerate with menthone, cineol, inactive pinene, and limonene. The oil is stimulant, stomachic, carminative, and antispasmodic. It is used for all pains in the alimentary canal, is combined with purgatives to prevent griping, and is used in the treatment of diarrhea and cholera as well as to disguise the taste of less palatable medicines.

Pennyroyal (*Mentha pulegium*) was named by Pliny because of its reputation for driving away fleas, the Latin word for flea being "pulex."

Unlike the other mints, pennyroyal creeps on the ground forming a dense, low mat. An infusion of the herb is an old-fashioned, and still effective, remedy for colds and menstrual irregularities. It is carminative, diaphoretic, stimulant, and emmenagogic, used by herbalists for flatulence, nausea, stomach spasms, and hysteria.

It is, as its botanic name attests, excellent for getting rid of fleas. I rub my dog with the crushed leaves and put a strong decoction in the water when I mop the floors.

All the mints are easy to cultivate, all do well in rich loamy soil, and they like plenty of water. They spread quickly from creeping rootstalks, and confining them to their allotted space is a greater problem than getting them started. They are an addition to any garden for beauty of foliage and for fragrance, which pervades the air, and for attractive white, pink, and lavender blossoms. Their fresh taste is both healthy and appetizing.

Besides spearmint, peppermint, and pennyroyal, there are four more mints that will add interest and variety to the garden. Orange and lemon mint have a special fragrance which makes them delicious tea herbs. The round-leaved apple mint and the low-growing, tiny-leaved Corsican mint are pretty and useful to put in a cool drink or to freeze in ice cubes.

The literature of the 19th century in the United States shows us that mint was a valued herb. In "The Country of the Pointed Firs," Sarah Orne Jewett describes the garden of Mrs. Todd, a practicing herbalist and lover of plants: ". . . the sea breezes blew into the low end window of the house laden with . . . balm, and sage and borage and mint, wormwood and southernwood."

The Peoples' Common Sense Medical Advisor [1895] recommends peppermint for the treatment of spasms, colic, and hysteria. The infusion, it says, "may be used freely." Spearmint it recommends for "its dieuretic and febrifuge virtues." Pennyroyal should be "used freely in the form of a worm infusion, promotes perspiration and excites the menstrual discharge. A large draught of the infusion should be taken at bed-time."

NETTLE

STINGING NETTLE	*Urtica dioica* L.
SMALL NETTLE	*U. urens* L.
	URTICACEAE

Nettles, despite their perfect adaptation to every square mile of the United States, are not native to North America. The first seeds were brought over from England by that indefatigable gardener, John Josselyn, testifying to their importance in the mother country.

The stinging nettle is perennial with a stem about three feet long. The downy, opposite leaves are tapering, deeply and evenly serrated, three

73

to five inches long and one to three inches across, covered with stinging, bristly hairs. The small, green flowers are arranged on branching
pyramids or "panicles," some erect (the male) and some hanging (the
female). Nettles prefer soil rich in nitrogen, and their presence in the
garden is a good indication of nitrogen content.

The nettle's chemical components include formic acid, mucilage,
ammonia, carbonic acid, and water.

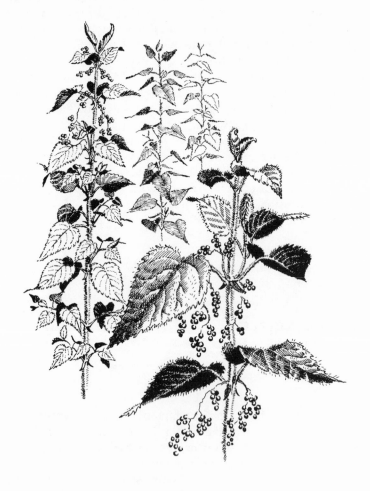

Nettle

Nettle is a potent herb, with many uses. Medicinally, it is diuretic, astringent, and tonic.

The stinging hairs on the leaves contain bicarbonate of ammonia, which does not survive heat; the cooked nettles, therefore, are edible.

The green herb, boiled in a strong salt solution, will curdle milk and is used instead of rennet in home-made cheeses.

Breathing in the burning dried leaves of nettle is a home treatment for asthma and bronchial problems.

A tea made from three or four leaves in an infusion of one and one-half cups of boiling water is a spring tonic and blood purifier.

It is antiscorbutic. The same infusion may be applied locally to treat burns. The fresh juice arrests bleeding and, diluted half and half with water, is an astringent gargle.

The leaves can be used to treat rheumatism, sciatica, and infertility. They are recommended as an addition to the diet of diabetics. Used raw and applied directly to the rheumatic pain area, they increase circulation and draw out pain. The painful area should be oiled with olive or safflower oil before applying nettle leaves.

When the Romans brought nettles to England, they did so because they had heard that the climate was miserably cold. They whacked their bodies with branches of nettle to increase circulation.

A recipe that dates back to the Roman occupation of England recommends nettles "salted in oil" be rubbed on the body to keep out the cold.

Young, fresh leaves, gathered when they are not more than six inches long, may be used as a pot herb. Put them in a colander, wash thoroughly under running water, drain, and cook covered, without adding any more water than clings to the leaves. Chop, add butter and pepper to taste.

Nettle is a good addition to a vegetable casserole. To a cup and one-half of cooked rice add equal amounts of scalded chopped nettles, broccoli, leeks (or onions), parsley, and basil to taste. Dribble sea salt and pepper on top.

Nettle fibers have been used, like flax, for textiles in many parts of the world. During World War I, Germany collected over two million kilograms which were used to make army uniforms.

Like many herbs which have been prescribed successfully for hundreds of years, nettles appear in many old rhymes.

> *If they would eat nettles in March*
> *And drink mugwort in May,*
> *So many fine maidens*
> *Would not go to the clay.*

Another old adage used to be recited while ridding oneself of a nettle sting, had one approached the plant incautiously.

> *Nettle in, dock out*
> *Dock rub nettle out.*

Burdock, like nettle, grows everywhere; following this maxim should not be difficult.

When cut and allowed to dry, nettles may be mixed with hay and fed to cattle. This will increase the yield of milk. Dried, powdered, and fed to hens, it will increase laying.

Flies dislike nettles, and a bunch hung on the outside of the kitchen door will keep them away.

The seeds mixed with food will increase the glossiness of both dogs' and horses' coats.

The nettle, or "wergulu" in the old Wessex dialect of the tenth century, was one of the nine sacred herbs, along with mugwort, plantain, watercress, chamomile, crab apple, chervil, and fennel.

Urtica urens, the small nettle, is an annual, six to eighteen inches high, with stinging bristly branches and thin oval leaves, deeply serrate on rather long petioles. Flower clusters are about the same length as the petioles, or shorter, the flowers androgynous (having both staminate and pistillate flowers in the same inflorescence).

Urtica urens and many of the fifty species of *Urtica* can be used in the same way suggested for *Urtica dioica*.

PARSLEY

PARSLEY	*Petroselinum crispum* (Mill.) Nym. ex. A. W. HILL
	UMBELLIFERAE

Parsley, ruled by Mars, belongs to a valuable family of herbs which includes anise, dill, fennel, coriander, and caraway, all of which are aromatic, carminative, condiment, and stimulant—caraway also being galactagogue.

Parsley was revered by the Greeks and Romans and is used today in every country of the world.

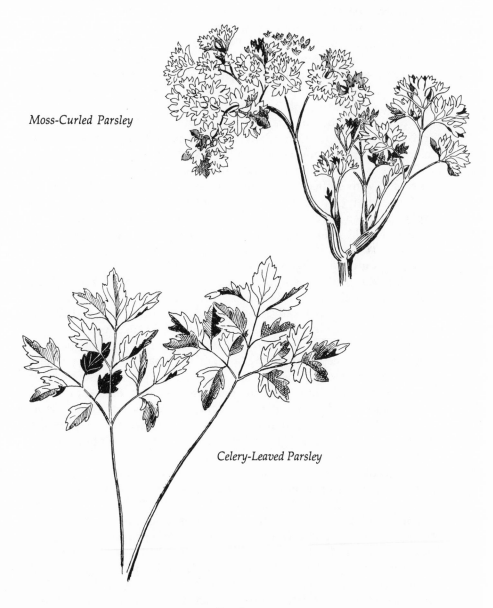

Moss-Curled Parsley

Celery-Leaved Parsley

Parsley

Two varieties of parsley should be represented in our gardens, the moss-curled because of its beauty, and the Italian or celery-leaved because it is hardier in very cold winters. Both varieties have the same constituents: up to three percent of volatile oil consisting of apiol (parsley camphor) and a terpene resin, fixed oil, and mucilage.

Leaves, seeds, and root have medicinal value in the treatment of diseases of the bladder and kidneys (gravel, stones, congestion, and jaundice), and for rheumatism, arthritis, and sciatica. Parsley is high in iron content and rich in vitamins A, B, and C and trace minerals. The bruised leaves, applied externally, are used by herbalists, alone or with celandine, comfrey, and red clover, to dispel tumors.

Parsley is easy to cultivate. It is a biennial, but self-seeds for years in a rich soil with sufficient moisture and a little shade.

The seeds try our patience if we wait for them to come up, as is explained by an old country saying that parsley "goes nine times to the devil and back" before it appears above the ground. Ideally, "it should be sown on Good Friday, under a rising moon." Sow four times as much as you need to "give the devil his due."

I plant the seeds by sprinkling them on top of well-worked, sifted soil, covered only by wet newspaper held down by stones at the corners. I water the paper daily, or twice a day if it dries out, and do not remove it until the leaves break through the soil beneath it.

An old superstition warns that it is unlucky to transplant parsley. Because of the exceptionally long tap root, it probably *is* unlucky unless you have a truly emerald thumb. I usually dig up a very small plant from my second or third planting, put it in a pot that looks far too big, and am always surprised at how quickly it branches out and fills it. Parsley, like all plants potted for winter kitchen use, will adapt to the change with less shock if it is watered with a weak solution of seaweed—one tablespoon to a gallon of water.

The second-year parsley should be cut back as soon as the flower stalks shoot up. This will cause it to bush out and will provide you with cuttings until well after the first snow.

Parsley was so well thought of in sixteenth-century England that William Turner said if it were thrown into fish ponds it would "heal the sick fishes therin."

Eat parsley raw in salads, make tea of the seeds, put finely chopped leaves on baked potatoes, in soups and egg dishes, in home-made mayonnaise, sour cream, and yogurt to use as a topping for vegetables. Mix it with cottage cheese as a side dish and make a parsley butter for open-faced summer sandwiches. Parsley may be substituted for basil in recipes for pesto sauce.

Parsley Butter

To one cup of sweet or lightly salted butter at room temperature, add finely chopped fresh parsley leaves until smooth and green flecked. Cover with foil and keep in the refrigerator until needed. This makes a nice topping for broiled fish or green beans.

Plants of the moss-curled variety make a handsome border in the herb garden or kitchen plot. In Athens, in the old section of the city called "The Plaka," parsley and basil are seen in every tiny garden, on window sills and in doorways.

SAGE

SAGE	*Salvia officinalis* L.
PINEAPPLE SAGE	*S. elegans* Vahl.
CLARY SAGE	*S. sclarea* L.
	LABIATAE

Sage is governed by Jupiter, the benevolent planet that sponsors nutrition and genial living. A native of the Mediterranean, it grows wild from the southern coast of Spain to Marseilles and on both the Mediterranean and Adriatic coasts of Italy. It establishes itself happily in thin soils of limestone foundation and grows profusely in Croatia and Dalmatia. We often see little jars on the condiment shelves of food stores labeled "Dalmatian Rubbed Sage."

Its official name, *Salvia*, is from the Latin verb, "salvare," to save, proof that this herb has been valued since Roman times and before. The old saying, *Cur moriatur homo cui Salvia crescit in horto?* or "Why should a man die when he has sage in his garden?" is certainly an expression of confidence in the medicinal and preventive powers of sage.

79

An old tradition called for planting rue next to sage. It is believed that the bitter herb would protect the valued medicinal one from the depredations of toads. In my garden, both plants seem able to protect themselves, and I use them both extensively. I put chopped fresh sage on buttered whole-wheat bread as a open-faced sandwich, mix the leaves into softened cheddar cheese, sprinkle them on eggs "buerre noir," and infuse the fresh or dried leaves (standard brew) for a delicious tea, alone or in combination with other blander herbs. The Chinese at one

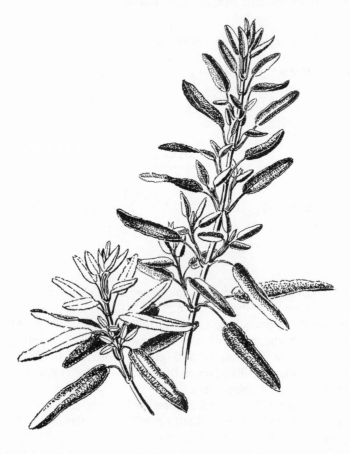

Sage

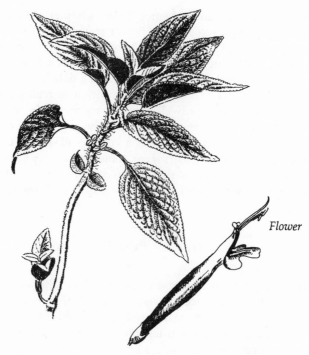

Flower

Pineapple Sage

time thought so highly of sage tea that one pound of it was worth three pounds of their own tea in trade with the Dutch.

Sage is a hardy perennial even in northern Vermont and will continue to grow well for about four years. I start a few new plants from seed every spring, planting them outdoors in the garden as soon as the soil has warmed from its winter cover of snow. Sage plants are low-growing, and their opposite, oblong leaves are olive-green with a pebbly texture. The flowers are red-violet (on my plants), but the garden sage, *Salvia officinalis*, varies greatly depending on the amount of sun and lime content of the soil. There are over five hundred varieties of sage. They grow throughout the tropical and temperate zones and many of them have medicinal and culinary value.

Salvia sclarea, clary sage, belongs in every garden for its beauty as well as the fact that it makes a pleasant liquor. (See instructions for home-made liquers under Lemon Balm, Chapter VII.) It grows much taller than garden sage and the flower stalks grace any bouquet.

Pineapple sage, *S. elegans*, is not hardy in Vermont but can be brought indoors for the winter. Fragrant, with deep pink blossoms, it has the fragrance of a true ripe pineapple. It makes a delicious tea, and the fresh leaves are a healthy and appetizing addition to fruit punches.

Garden sage and speedwell (*Veronica officinalis*) in equal parts make a good general tea for everyday preventive use and social enjoyment.

The active ingredient of sage is a volatile oil. It also contains tannin and resin. It is stimulant, astringent, tonic, carminative, and disinfectant.

Gerard wrote, "Sage is singularly good for the head and brain, it quickeneth the senses and memory, strengtheneth the sinews. . . ."

Recipe for Eggs Buerre Noir

Fry eggs gently in a buttered, covered skillet. Remove when done to a warm platter and place in a warm (200 degree) oven. Put a lump of butter for each egg in the skillet and cook until brown. Just as it reaches the desired color, add 1/4 teaspoon of cider vinegar for each egg. Mix and spoon over eggs; sprinkle with finely minced fresh or dry sage.

Sage and sea salt rubbed together are a good homemade dentifrice which removes tartar and whitens the teeth. A mouthwash of sage, rosemary, peppermint, and comfrey made by infusion (double strength standard brew) with the addition of a tablespoon of natural cider vinegar and honey will keep the gums healthy and the breath sweet. Fenugreek can be substituted for honey, as it is also disinfectant and sweet. It is often used commercially as a maple syrup flavor.

Sage has always been an ingredient in traditional stuffing for turkey and in sausage. It adds not only taste but also built-in prevention against discomfort from overeating or indigestion.

If you plant sage in your garden, remember that after you have harvested all the perfect leaves for drying you can scatter the yellow, bruised, or dusty lower leaves along the rows to be tilled into the soil for protection against nematodes (worms) which might be seeking winter refuge in your garden. Sage is used in this manner, as a soil disinfectant, by owners of fruit orchards and tomato farms in Mexico.

SALAD BURNET

SALAD BURNET   *Sanguisorba officinalis* L.
ROSACEAE

Salad burnet is one of those endearing little herbs whose presence in our garden is so decorative, and whose uses as food and medicine so

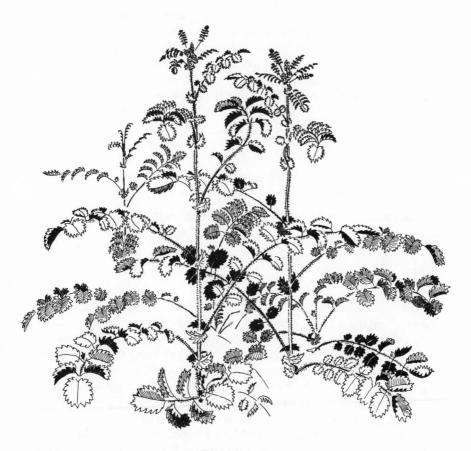

Salad Burnet

pleasant that, while it is not one of the most important additions to our table and pharmacopeia, it is, nevertheless, a minor blessing.

The small, acutely serrated, bright-green leaflets grow on spreading, wiry stems in pairs of five to ten. They have a mild cucumber flavor, and like cucumber, are cooling to the system. The flower heads never actually bear open florets, but resemble a pointed strawberry or a diminutive scarlet pine cone. The tufted stigmas are somewhat drooping.

Burnet grew in all the old European herb gardens and was an early immigrant to America. Its name, *Sanguisorba*, is derived from "sanguis," blood, which gives us a clue to its ability to stanch blood flow from wounds. The plant is healing, tonic, styptic, and cooling.

The young leaves, cut up in salad, add their cucumber flavor and vitamin content. They are a nice addition to cottage cheese.

An infusion of leaves and flower heads (standard brew) is tonic and cooling as a tea, taken a cupful at a time, once or twice a day. This same infusion may be used externally to soothe a bad case of sunburn or any skin irritation.

SAVORY

SUMMER SAVORY	*Satureja hortensis* L.
WINTER SAVORY	*S. montana*
	LABIATAE

Culpepper says that savory is under the dominion of Mercury, the planet which makes connection between thought and action. It was used by Greeks and Romans, often combined with thyme, to flavor game, soups, and stuffings, much as it is today. Records show that it was used by the Saxons and was cultivated in the gardens of Charlemagne. Early English colonists brought it to this country; John Winthrop, Jr., ordered a half ounce of summer savory seed at two-pence and one ounce of winter savory at sixpence. We find reference to the savories in that most practical of garden books, Leonard Meager's 1682 *Art of Gardening,* which came to America from England. A much-used copy was in the library of Governor Winthrop of the Massachusetts Bay Colony.

Savory is carminative, expectorant, astringent, and stomachic. The

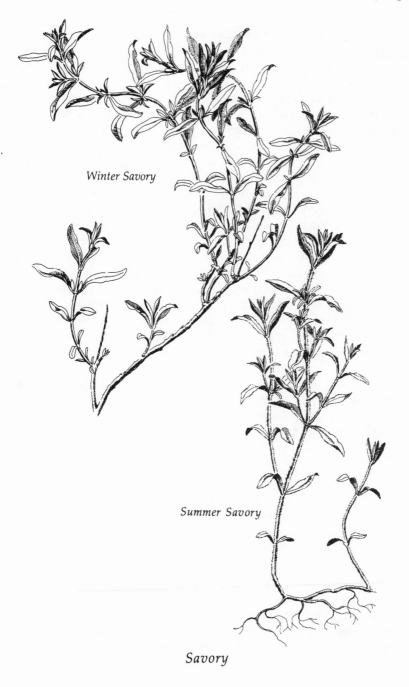

Winter Savory

Summer Savory

Savory

carminative effect of the savories make them the ideal condiment for cooking with beans and peas. A few of the leaves cooked with cabbage, cauliflower, and turnips will absorb the strong odor usually associated with these vegetables.

A tea (standard brew) is a safe home remedy for intestinal disorders, and its astringent qualities recommend savory as a cure for diarrhea. The infusion may also be used as a gargle for sore throat.

Summer savory is an annual which often self-sows in the garden. It is hardy, and the seeds seem to grow into strong plants after freezing in the ground. The seeds may be sown as soon as the ground can be worked. The erect, slender stems attain a height of from fifteen to twenty inches in my garden. The blunt, oblong, nearly linear leaves taper to short petioles on the main stem. Labiate, pale pinkish-lavender flowers form in the axils of the leaves in mid-summer. Usually two cuttings of the leafy tips can be made before the blossoms appear. When blossoms do, the plant should be pulled up to dry for winter use.

Winter savory, *Satureja montana,* is a hardy, low, much-branched, shrubby perennial, which can be used as a decorative plant on a rocky ledge or in a raised bed. The leaves are a sleek, dark green, the flowers paler than the summer savory—nearly white. It has all the culinary and medicinal value of its sister annual and once started can be increased by root division or layering.

Virgil recommended planting savory to attract honey bees. Visiting bees seem interested in my plants, and I have discovered that the leaves will take the sting out of their inadvertent bites, if rubbed on them immediately.

SWEET CICELY

SWEET CICELY *Myrrhis odorata* (L.) Scop.
UMBELLIFERAE

The long black seeds of sweet cicely are used in confections, the feathery leaves in soups and salads. Like anise, which it resembles in fragrance and taste, it is carminative and stomachic.

Sweet cicely is a very handsome plant in the garden. Its lacy-branched leaves fan out from the stem, and its small white flowers add accent against the deeper green and pink-to-purple flowers of other herbs.

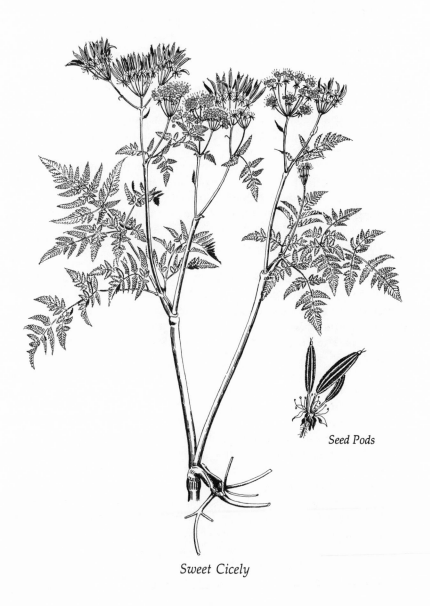

Seed Pods

Sweet Cicely

VERVAIN

BLUE OR FALSE VERVAIN
("WILD HYSSOP")

Verbena hastata L.

VERBENACEAE

Vervain grows three to five feet high. The opposite leaves are lanceolate, thin, serrate to deeply incised dentate, three to six inches long. Deep blue-to-purplish flowers grow on long terminal pedicels. It is indigenous to North America and is found growing wild from the Atlantic seaboard to the Pacific coast.

Blue vervain is antiperiodic, diaphoretic, diuretic, tonic, vermifuge, and vulnerary. It has been used for more than thirty diseases, and among other valuable qualities it is a natural tranquilizer.

A warm infusion of either root, leaves, or flowers, taken every few hours, is helpful for colds and fevers, throat and chest congestion, and headache. A poultice of the bruised fresh leaves gives relief in cases of neuralgia and rheumatism.

Vervain was used by the American Indians to treat stomach ache; and one tribe, the Menominees, used it to clear up cloudy urine.[1] The early colonists soon assimilated the knowledge of its medical virtues because records show that army surgeons used it during the Revolutionary War. They described its action as "kind and beneficial."

Cotton Mather, in *The Angel of Bethesda*, recommended it for the treatment of consumption. Take "a convenient Quantity, make a strong Decoction. Then add unto the Decoction an equal Quantity of Honey; and boil them together into the Consistency of a syrup. Of this take now and then a spoonful."

This prescription of Cotton Mather is interesting because of the instructions to "take now and then a spoonful." These can be applied to the herbal recipes in this book. Except where it is specifically stated that a certain herb may have specified results if taken in large quantities, it is not necessary to be a precision chemist to put together safe and useful herbal remedies for home use. This is the positive side. It must be added that "instant" cures should not be expected except in specifically stated

---

[1] Virgil J. Vogel, *American Indian Medicine*. Norman: University of Oklahoma Press, 1970.

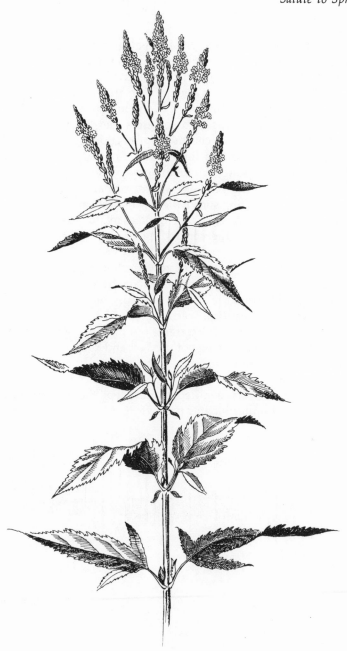

Vervain

cases. Herbs that are listed as "alterative" gradually restore the healthy balance of the body and must be taken over a long period of time.

The European *Verbena officinalis* was used by priests for sacrifices, and the name verbena was a general Roman term for altar plants, vervain in particular. It was included in the lustral water (used in rites of purification) by the druids, and sorcerers had great faith in it. It was worn around the neck as a charm for protection against headaches and the bite of serpents. But as the conscientious Gerard tells us "many odde old wives fables are written of vervaine tending to witchcraft and sorcery, which you may read elsewhere, for I am not willing to trouble your eares with reporting such trifles, as honest eares abhorre to heare."

A former use for vervain that is pleasant to "the eares" was as a token of good faith in the concluding of treaties—no man of honest intentions would enter a parley without it.

For medicinal use, the stalks of vervain should be cut just as the buds begin to adorn the curving panicles. I have transplanted vervain to my garden where it grows well and self-seeds freely. As John Burroughs said, "Vervain is a beautiful weed. . . ."

Herbs are natural insect deterrents but only vervain seems to attract grasshoppers. I take advantage of this fact and keep a generous planting of them well back from the edge of the garden. In dry summers when grasshoppers become a menace to the appearance of flowers and vine crops, this outpost acts as a decoy and keeps the marauders chewing happily until a rain terminates their visit.

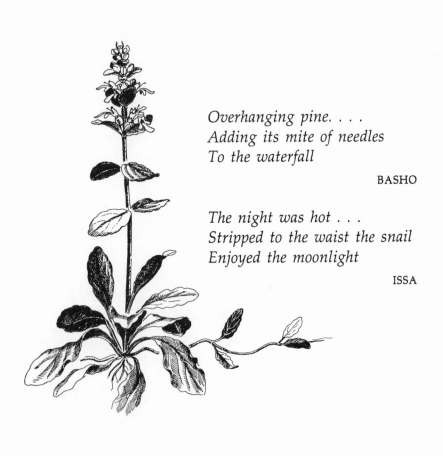

Overhanging pine. . . .
Adding its mite of needles
To the waterfall

BASHO

The night was hot . . .
Stripped to the waist the snail
Enjoyed the moonlight

ISSA

VII

Summer:
Gourmet Gardening

One morning the sun, high above the river, sucks up white ribbons of mist and draws them into the cumulus clouds that hang motionless in a bland cobalt sky. Brilliant sunshine streaks in through a south window and impartially spotlights a hand-blown goblet and minute particles of dust vibrating in the warm air.

Something has changed since yesterday. Barefoot, I walk into the kitchen and flip the page of a wall calendar from May to June.

Suddenly it is summer. In the garden low-creeping mother-of-thyme extends tiny green tentacles over the flagstone path. The little whorls around the stem are showing violet buds. It is time to cut the first batch of stiff little branches for drying.

In Tangier, while visiting my *comadre* (mother of my Spanish son-in-law), I learned to rub dried thyme into roasted coriander and sesame seeds. Add a little sea salt to this mixture, and you will have a delicious sprinkle for buttered slices of rye, whole-wheat, or French bread. Put them in the sun just long enough to melt the butter. Serve with a large bowl of summer salad. Use your own combinations for this and try one of my favorites:

Three kinds of lettuce: ruby leaf, salad bowl, oak leaf
Very thin slices of young zucchini and onions
Shredded comfrey, violet, and nasturtium leaves
Several sprigs of purslane
A few sections of fresh orange or grapefruit
One or two Jerusalem artichokes sliced very thin

Make a dressing of olive oil, fresh lemon juice, sea salt mixed with finely chopped dill weed, basil, and tarragon, two garlic cloves put through a press, and a little freshly ground black pepper.

Bon appetit, and remember that the conquering Roman legions ate coriander seeds and garlic on bread as their daily rations when away from home.

Deep red stems of English peppermint begin to distinguish it from the other square-stemmed mints: orange, apple, lemon, and spearmint. All these fragrant varieties can be used in jellies, sauces, as a piquant addition to a green salad, or crushed in the bottom of a frosted mint julep glass. An idiosyncratic member of the family is Corsican mint. It hugs the ground more closely than woolly thyme, its minute, round, green leaves huddled together so closely that they seem stemless. Stoop down and rub your finger across it and be surprised that anything so tiny could have such a strong fragrance. It is hardy even in the coldest winter. As soon as the snow melts, the little leaves begin to spread over the ground.

Mints can be used in cooking the most prosaic vegetables, turning them into festive dish.

Minted Carrots

Steam young carrots (two handfuls) for seven minutes. In a skillet melt two tablespoons butter, one tablespoon maple syrup, one tablespoon rum, one tablespoon finely chopped mint (orange or peppermint). Add the carrots, which should be just barely tender. Warm all together for three minutes. Serve with a sprig of mint on top.

Carob Mint Pudding

ໜ

Melt, stirring constantly, four tablespoons carob in two cups milk. Add three-quarters cup honey. When dissolved, remove from fire and add three lightly beaten egg yolks. Reheat, stirring constantly, until mixture begins to thicken. Remove from fire, cool, add one tablespoon finely chopped peppermint and three stiffly beaten egg whites. Chill. Serve with whipped cream to which one teaspoon crème de menthe has been added.

Crème de Menthe

ໜ

To one bottle of vodka (i.e., 4/5 quart) add one cup crushed spearmint or peppermint, one and one-half cups honey, and a few drops of green vegetable coloring. Put in a tightly closed glass jar, shake well once a week and allow to stand for one month.

The same basic recipe can be used to make liqueurs from lemon balm (melissa), anise, sweet cicely, sage and lovage.

A few minutes spent out of doors, walking in a lush summer garden—gathering textured lettuce leaves, fragrant basil and dill, savory and green beans, beets, carrots, and broccoli, cut when they are exactly the right size (and only what we feel like eating this particular day)— is a more satisfying experience than getting in a car and driving through carbon-monoxide-scented air to buy vegetables and herbs that may be many miles and days away from their source. Our selection is based on what is available as well as what we want.

Perhaps it is not possible for us all to grow our own food this year. But there will be other years. And we can all make changes in our lives if we begin to connect the food we eat with our state of health and well being.

Summer is the time of year when we see the maturity of plants all around us, when gradual development has reached logical fruition, when the clue to the present is traceable in the past.

Lest we be accused of nostalgia, let us face the fact that much "modern" knowledge is simply rediscovering the wisdom of the past. The Egyptians used cabbage seeds to prevent intoxication. Today cabbage juice is being used to treat alcoholism. As recorded in the Ebers Papyrus, they also used thyme to cure fungus infection. Today thyme is being used in Spanish hospitals as a wound disinfectant. Garlic, which we know today is a natural antibiotic, was so highly valued by the Egyptians that fifteen pounds of it was the going rate for an able-bodied slave.

Dioscorides wrote of the *Salix alba* (white willow) as an anodyne. Aspirin (acetyl salicylic acid) is on every drug counter today.

As we watch our summer garden leaf out to lush maturity, we understand why green has always been known as the color of healing. Light cerulean blue shades into violet and indigo as the evening sky above the garden darkens at sunset. These are the colors associated with spirituality. Mid-summer, for many people, is vacation time, but even those who choose winter as the season away from work patterns usually select a locale where they can contemplate blue skies and green vistas.

June twenty-first, the summer solstice, or St. John's Eve, is the longest day in the year. At noontime the Sun, exactly ninety degrees between the vernal and autumnal equinox, seems to stand still before it retraces its path down the heavenly arc. As herb gardeners, we have a link with the public bonfires which glowed in small villages all over sixteenth-century Europe to celebrate St. John's Eve. Garlands of mugwort (*Artemisia vulgaris*) and vervain (*Verbena officinalis*) were worn by young and old, who watched the flames through sprays of larkspur which they believed would protect their eyesight throughout the year. As they returned home, each one threw his garland of herbs into the dying flames, asking the fire to burn away his ill luck.

The American Indians used *Artemisias* to line their sweat lodges in their purification ceremonies. Today we take *Artemisia absinthium* as a tea to purify our systems in the spring. In summer we use it as one of our important insecticides.

Fresh or dried leaves can be chopped and placed in a circle around young cabbage plants when first set out in the garden. The bitter taste discourages insects. Fresh leaves, finely chopped and mixed with coarse sand or sharp pebbles, should be kept around the plants all summer to discourage slugs whose bellies are vulnerable to abrasive surfaces. This will protect strawberry beds from slugs and young green beans from cutworms.

An herbal spray that protects against insect marauders is made by chopping equal parts of wormwood, tansy, rue, hyssop, and pennyroyal with a clove of chopped garlic. Add to a quart of water, let it come to a boil, and steep it for thirty minutes. Strain, add another quart of water and spray on the plants. It is harmless to children, animals, and birds, but insects find its strong scent unpleasant.

A happy summer marriage of herb and vegetable is that between savory and green bean. It gives flavor to the beans and prevents gas from forming in the stomach.

When cooking dried beans, split peas, or lentils, the flavor can be made delicious and intriguing by the addition of fresh or dried savory, marjoram, thyme, and basil, as well as one bay leaf and a grated carrot.

The wealth of flavors and appetizing odors possible with fresh herbs makes summer cooking a culinary adventure.

My summer soup and zucchini pancake recipes may start you off on your own gourmet garden fantasy.

Adele's Summer Soup

Two handfuls each of sorrel and purslane
One handful watercress
A few leaves each of basil and lovage, a sprig of tarragon
One-half cup of minced chervil
One clove garlic, crushed
One hot red pepper, minced
Two large onions, chopped
Two large potatoes, chopped fine
Two tablespoons butter
Four cups vegetable soup stock
One cup cream

Put butter in a large iron pot. Stir in sorrel, purslane, watercress, basil, lovage, and tarragon, garlic, hot pepper, and onion. Stir until herbs are wilted and onion transparent. Add finely chopped potato and stir one minute. Add vegetable soup stock and simmer thirty minutes. Add one teaspoon sea salt and one cup cream. Serve hot or chilled with finely minced chervil on top of each serving.

Adele's Zucchini Pancakes

ta

Three small or one and one-half large zucchini, grated
A few finely chopped basil leaves and marjoram and savory sprigs
One-half cup grated cheddar cheese
One cup whole-wheat flour, unsifted
One teaspoon salt
One teaspoon baking powder
One lightly beaten egg
Dash of cayenne pepper
Enough milk and/or yogurt to make a thick batter

Combine all ingredients and fry in a lightly greased iron skillet until golden brown on both sides. Serve with one-half cup yogurt and one-half cup sour cream, well blended.

For dessert, serve a tall glass of comfrey pineapple drink (see page 36) with a scoop of lime sherbet in it.

Lime Sherbet

ta

One-half cup lime juice
One cup water
Three-quarters cup honey
One cup heavy cream, whipped
Two stiffly beaten egg whites

Combine the first three ingredients and warm in pan until honey has dissolved. Remove from fire, cool, and add whipped cream and stiffly beaten egg whites. Pour into ice container and freeze. When partially frozen, take out, beat in a bowl, return to container and finish freezing.

Herbs, always versatile, make gifts that appeal to sight, scent, and taste.

A "tussie-mussie" is a bouquet concocted of fragrant herbs surrounded by a lace paper doily and tied with ribbon. One rosebud is the traditional center, but a carnation, or gilly flower as it was called in the days when the tussie-mussie was popular, may be substituted as may be an English daisy (*Bellis perennis*). The center flower is surrounded by fragrant herbs:

rosemary, lavender, scented geranium, lemon verbena, lemon balm, valerian, or any of the mint family, to make a symmetrical bouquet.

Cut just enough out of the center of the doily to have it fit snugly around the stems. Wrap them with foil and tie with a ribbon. This sweet-smelling and unusual gift can rise to many occasions: birthday, bon voyage, or to send on-stage to a performing artist friend.

Herb jellies can be made in summer and kept on the shelf for Christmas or house-guest gifts throughout the year. The basic recipe can be used with fresh herbs in your garden or those bought at a local farmer's market.

Herb Jellies

This basic recipe can be used successfully with sage, rosemary, tarragon, marjoram, basil, lemon verbena, melissa, and anise.

Wash two quarts of ripe crab apples (or tart apples), cut up, unpeeled, and uncored. Just barely cover with water in a heavy pan and cook until very soft. Empty into a jelly bag and let drip overnight. Measure juice, and for each cup allow one tablespoon cider vinegar, three-quarters cup sugar or honey, and three sprigs of an herb. Sometimes two or three herbs can be combined to produce a delicious but indefinable flavor.

Boil the crab-apple juice with the fresh herb, sugar or honey, and vinegar. If sugar is used, it should be heated in a flat pan in the oven before adding to the juice, which should be boiled for five minutes before the addition of the sugar. Boil the juice until it jells easily. To test, spoon out a little on a cold saucer. If it thickens quickly, it is done. If you have a food thermometer, bring the juice to two hundred and twenty degrees. Pour into hot, sterilized jelly jars. Allow to cool a few minutes and cover the top with melted paraffin. A fresh leaf of the herb may be put in the jelly if you like. In this case, pour an ounce of the jelly in the jar, put in the herb leaf, allow to set a minute, then fill the jar.

In making mint jelly, use the same recipe but boil a large handful of the mint with the crab-apple juice for ten minutes, then strain and continue boiling until the jelly stage is reached. To give mint jelly the expected green color, add a tablespoon of raw spinach juice or a few drops of green vegetable coloring.

99

Herb vinegars are less time-consuming than jellies and are also sure to be appreciated as gifts.

Herb Vinegars
ও

Fill a quart jar three-quarters full of fresh tarragon, rosemary, or basil leaves. Bring just to boiling point enough apple cider or wine vinegar to fill the jar. Pour, hot, over the herb and fill the jar. Cover tightly and allow to stand for two weeks, shaking the jar every few days. Strain and bottle.

Garlic vinegar is made the same way, but eight garlic cloves, crushed, are put in the quart jar before the hot vinegar is added.

The following recipe for dandelion wine, besides its fine flavor and genial effect, has another distinct advantage. Your self-image will expand to include "frugal homemaker" and "gourmet hostess" once the golden-hued bottles are on your shelf.

Dandelion Wine
ও

Eight gallons dandelion flower heads
Four gallons water
Five oranges, quartered
Two lemons, quartered
Two packages dry yeast
Crushed ginger root (optional)
Seven pounds sugar

Collect the dandelions on a bright sunny day when the vitamins you absorb from "Solis Invictus" will compensate for any backache involved. Children under ten years make good companions for this safari as they are closer to the ground than you are and normally enthusiastic about expeditions, especially if a hint is dropped that there may be cookies later.

Spread newspapers out on the grass, when you return home with your loot, and empty the dandelions on them. This will give the insects a chance to crawl away before you take the flowers inside to wash and put in a crock. Once they are in the crock, pour the four gallons of boiling water over them, cover, and wait twenty-four hours. Strain into a large enamel canning pot, add oranges, lemons, and ginger root. Boil thirty minutes, strain, add sugar, dissolve. Pour into crock. When cooled to lukewarm, stir in the yeast which has been dissolved in two tablespoons of the liquid. Cover and wait until it stops "working," or bubbling. This will take about ten days or a little longer, depending on the temperature.

When the working has stopped, siphon into gallon jugs, cork loosely, and wait one month before decanting wine into quart bottles. The wine will be excellent by Thanksgiving. You may want to sample a bottle by Labor Day just to see if you have a good year.

CUTTING HERBS FOR DRYING

The proper time for drying herbs is when they are at their peak which is just as the flower buds begin to open. This is when the essential essence is most potent, when the energy that has been stored in the root all winter has gradually crept up the stem to produce foliage and blossoms—the extravaganza of summer. Soon the flower will produce seed, the "herb-bearing seed" of Genesis within which is carried the unchanging paradigm of next year's plant.

There is another reason for not waiting until the flowering is complete, a reason analogous to shopping for summer merchandise at the beginning of the season. When we find perfect specimens of herbs, we are not the only ones in the market for nature's benefits. Insects, birds, bees, and animals have the same instinct for preserving and restoring health that we have. But we need not feel guilty about getting there first; they have a much larger cruising range than we have.

Choose a warm, sunny day and wait until the dew has dried, for moist foliage is likely to become moldy. Cut the stems just above ground level and divide them into loose bunches, about a handful to each bunch. Tie the stems with string or strips of cloth, hang them, blossom down, out of direct sun (which would discolor the leaves) in a room or shed with cross-ventilation. Print tags with the name of the herb and the date, and attach them securely to the string. This will save confusion when you are ready to bottle the herbs, which, when dry, with curled leaves, are not always easy to recognize even with the aid of scent.

Heavy-leaved herbs with thick veining take longer to dry than small, thin-leaved plants, sometimes up to three weeks if the weather is rainy or damp. If you can predict that you will be very busy by the time the herbs are ready to bottle, hang them up, covered with large paper bags, the open end tied around the stem, the other end cut out for ventilation. This will protect the herbs from dust, and you can rub them down and bottle them when you have more time.

When the herbs are perfectly dry, hold them over a large bowl and rub the leaves and flowers off the stems. Then cut the stems in small bits. Use glass jars, tins, or ceramic containers for storage, but be sure the lids fit securely. Label each herb at once with name and date of bottling. (See Chapter VIII.)

Another system for drying herbs is to place them on layers of screen or muslin stretched over frames.

In either case, if you have a free day and the herbs are not bone dry, you can finish the process by setting your oven at two hundred degrees and turning it off when it has reached that temperature. Put the herbs, spread out on a cookie sheet, in the oven for about ten to twenty minutes.

Herbs used for flavoring only may be kept for two years; those used medicinally should be replaced every year. Tossing out unused herbs is not so wasteful as it sounds. What is left the next summer should be sprinkled around garden plants, dug into the soil, or added to the compost pile. Wormwood, southernwood, mugwort, tansy, rue, and hyssop all have specific value in the garden as insect repellents.

Parsley and basil should be handled in a different way than most herbs. Dip them quickly in and out of boiling, sea-salted water. Shake well until almost dry; then cut into small pieces and spread evenly on a cookie sheet. Place in an oven at the lowest possible temperature, or heat the oven first to two hundred degrees and then turn it off and place the cookie sheet inside. This method retains the color and taste.

Basil, parsley, marjoram, savory, and thyme can all be quick-frozen for winter use. Small bags with a combination of herbs can be frozen and later tossed, still frozen, into a winter soup. Experiment, try your own combinations. Several that you might like to try are: thyme, marjoram, and calendula florets; savory, marjoram, and basil; lovage, thyme, and basil.

Roots should be scrubbed thoroughly before drying. Use a stiff brush, and if this does not get them perfectly clean, scrape with a sharp knife.

Large roots and barks may be cut in thin slices before they are placed on a screen to dry. The process can be speeded up by placing the sliced roots or the barks in a warm, not hot, oven. They may also be placed on the sill of a slightly open window to air-dry.

Seeds dry best if allowed to remain on the stem. Put a fine mesh or cheesecloth bag around the seed head so as not to lose any that may fall off or be gobbled up by a visiting bird.

Ancient people who lived closer to the earth than we do today and were far more observant to the growth, health, and decline of plants divided herbs into groups that were "ruled" by certain planets. If you would like to experiment with cutting your herbs when the ruling planet of each is in a favorable position here is the list.

The Sun rules: burnet, celandine, centaury, chamomile, chickory, eyebright, marigold, mistletoe, pimpernel, rosemary, saffron, St. John's-wort, viper's bugloss.

The Moon rules: adder's tongue, chickweed, cleavers (goose-grass), loosestrife, privet, purslane, watercress, white poppy, white rose, willow.

Mars rules: basil, broom, hawthorne, the lesser celandine, stonecrop, thistle.

Mercury rules: dill, fennel, hazel, honeysuckle, marjoram, mulberry, parsley, southernwood, vervain.

Jupiter rules: agrimony, balm, betony, borage, chervil, chestnut, cinquefoil, dandelion, dock, houseleek, hyssop, red rose, sage, thistle.

Venus rules: alder, birch, blackberry, burdock, coltsfoot, cowslip, daisy, elder, fennel, foxglove, ground ivy, groundsel, mallow, meadowsweet, mint, mugwort, periwinkle, plantain, primrose, sanicle, sea holly, sorrel, tansy, thyme, valerian, vervain, violet, yarrow.

Saturn rules: bistort, comfrey, hemlock, henbane, ivy, moss, mullein, nightshade.

If you decide to investigate the claims of the ancients, be assured that you are in good company; Hippocrates, known as the father of medicine, believed in its truth and said that every physician should be trained in astrology.

Do I believe in the efficacy of this system of cutting plants? A fair question. Our neighborhood astrologer is off playing guitar with a country rock band, but I hope he will be back before the herb-drying season is here.

Now, in mid-summer it is time to sit in the sun and examine our backyard from a new point of reference—that of available and inexpensive vitamins. Perhaps we should first define vitamins, going a step beyond the concept that they must come in brown bottles with a neatly printed "ho-hum" on the label that says something like "the necessity for vitamin so-and-so in the human diet has not been established." For our laymen's purpose, a vitamin may be defined as an organic compound, neither protein, carbohydrate, nor fat, that is necessary for one or more body functions to maintain health and/or growth. Some of these vitamins cannot be manufactured by the body in sufficient quantities to maintain health, and must be obtained from food. If we subsist on "junk foods," we must greatly increase our daily intake of vitamins with the commercial variety. Our backyard patch of vitamin A may reveal alfalfa, comfrey, dandelion, lamb's quarters (*Chenopodium album* L.), parsley, and green and yellow vegetables.

Our vitamin B garden is less extensive; here we have only comfrey and fenugreek (*Trigonella foenum-graecum* L.), of which comfrey provides B_2 and B_{12} and fenugreek contains B and B_2. These are helpful in our diet, but for the complete gamut of vitamin B, eat two tablespoons of nutritional yeast every other day, added to whole grain or oat cereal, pancakes, muffins, vegetable loaf, or casseroles.

Vitamin C is better represented with parsley, green peppers, burdock, rose hips, elderberries, black currants, oregano, and purslane, that invader between the rows of everyone's garden. Purslane has even higher C content than rose hips, one of the best known sources of the C vitamin. Cayenne, horseradish, coriander, ground ivy, catnip, nettle, lamb's-quarters, and sorrel are also purveyors of vitamin C.

Vitamin E can be found in the garden only in very small quantities and only in anise, dandelion greens, and sunflower seeds. The principal source of vitamin E is wheat germ, available in D-alpha tocopheral. This is naturally derived, the vitamin in its most potent form.

Sitting, relaxed in a green summer garden, we feel so healthy that we give only a passing thought to needing vitamins other than the ones available to us in good, organically produced food. But we all sometimes find ourselves in situations where our choice of food is limited and an emergent situation may disturb our well-balanced life-style. This is not the place to give an analysis of commercially produced vitamins, but two books are listed in the Selected Bibliography, under the title of "Health," which will be helpful.

Sometimes after a rain, when the weeds in our garden suddenly sprint ahead of cultivated plants, we are subject to "midsummer blues." Before too zealously pulling out these intruders, read the descriptions of some of them in this chapter, and you will see that the "invaders" are as important to our health as plants we have put in and tended. Among these important but uninvited guests are: agrimony, burdock, celandine, evening primrose, ground ivy, hawkweed, jewel weed, mallows (*Malva sylvestris* and *Malva rotundifolia*), plantain, purslane, self-heal, and red clover.

More important in our search for health than any amount of weeding, watering, drying, or preserving is attunement with our garden, be it large or small, a little patch near the kitchen door or a few hanging baskets of herbs on the porch. Getting to know our herbs intimately makes us realize that their requirements and ours are basically the same— pure water, nourishing food, sunshine, and tender loving care. Like our plants, we are tied irrevocably to the eternal rhythm of seasons, long and short days, sunrise and nightfall. Tending and gathering for food and medicine reinforces our innate knowledge that we are capable of caring for ourselves, that our well-being is a matter of individual decision and responsibility.

AGRIMONY

AGRIMONY   *Agrimonia eupatoria* L.
("COCKLEBURR," "STICKLEWORT")

ROSACEAE

A search along country roads and in fields bordering farms will be rewarded by the sight of two- to three-feet high stalks of agrimony with long, narrow, much-cut leaves, seven to eight inches long near the ground, with terminal spikes of small yellow flowers. The deep green leaves are pinnate, divided up to the midrib into pairs of leaflets which get smaller as they go up the stalk, becoming only two to three inches at the top. The plant is a mild astringent, is tonic, diuretic, vulnerary, and antiscrofulous. It contains a bitter volatile oil and five percent tannin.

Pliny described agrimony as "an herb of princely authoritie"; Dioscorides recommended it for "them that have bad livers"; Green, in his *Universal Herbal,* said that it "cures the ague." It has been used in

105

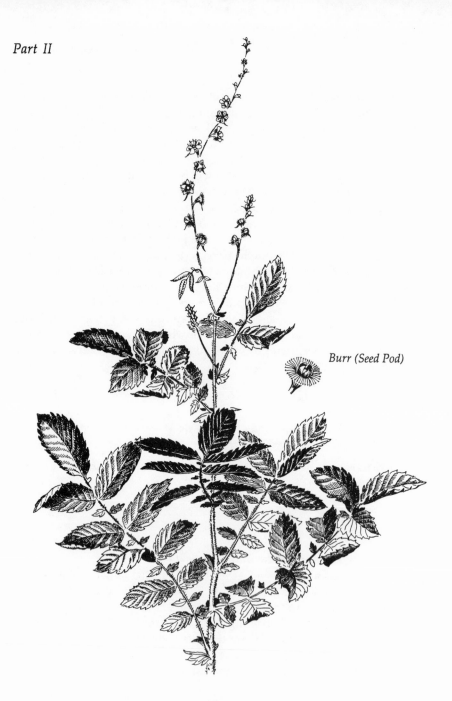

Burr (Seed Pod)

Agrimony

many countries as a spring tonic, alone or in combination with other herbs, to purify the blood. Sprains, bruises, stomach acidity, and diseases of the kidney, liver, and spleen respond well to agrimony.

In both infusion and decoction, herbalists use the whole herb in the treatment of coughs, diarrhea, dysentery, and intestinal colitis and as a post-operative tonic. It is used to get rid of pimples, skin blemishes, and all diseases of the blood. It has astringent action on the bladder and is used for the control of bed-wetting in older children. (Bed-wetting, however, is often a symptom of an emotional problem; thus, the cause must be dealt with as well as the overt behavior.)

I use agrimony frequently, in a strong infusion of the fresh or dried herb, to draw out splinters. Hold the affected part in a cup or bowl of the hot infusion for thirty minutes. The splinter will press out easily and painlessly. A combination of agrimony, mugwort, and vinegar is an excellent treatment for the pain of sciatica or muscular stiffness. Used as a mouthwash it removes tartar from the teeth. The infusion will also remove blackheads if allowed to remain on the spot for twenty minutes.

Dr. Daniel Smith, who practiced medicine in the first half of the nineteenth century wrote a book, *The Reformed Botanic and Indian Physician*, in which he recommended a decoction of agrimony to cure lunacy. As my friends and acquaintances seem reasonably sane, I have not had the opportunity to try this, but I do find agrimony useful for so many purposes that I have made a place for it in my garden. In Vermont it blooms late in the summer, and its small, bright, yellow blossoms, facing the August sky, are welcome suncatchers.

ANGELICA

ANGELICA   *Angelica archangelica* L.
                                                UMBELLIFERAE

A tall, ostentatiously handsome plant, angelica sends forth large, bright green, irregularly toothed leaves on hollow stems which rise four to nine feet. The large leaflets are arranged in groups of three, usually, but

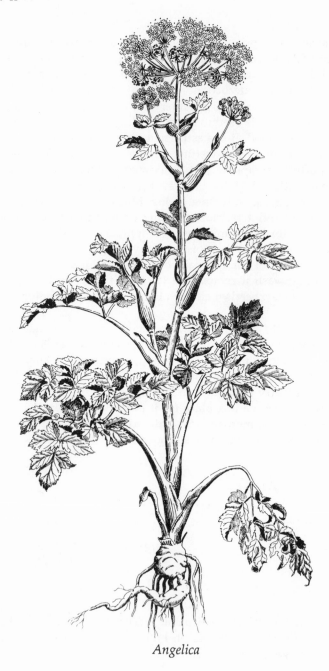

Angelica

sometimes up to five. Angelica is under the dominion of the sun, a self-sowing biennial which often takes three years to blossom; after this consummation the plants usually die. If the tops are cut before they flower the life of the plant can be prolonged several years. The roots are long and fusiform, and, like the stems and leaves, have a strong musky odor of juniper.

The plant has a long history of medicinal usefulness. During the Middle Ages it was used as protection against the plague. Culpepper said of Angelica: "In all epidemical diseases caused by Saturn that is as good a preservative as grows. It resists poison by defending and comforting the heart, blood, and spirits."

Roots, seeds and leaves are all used medicinally. Stems and seeds flavor confections, and dried leaves are used in the brewing of hop bitters.

The root of first year angelica plants, dug in autumn, should be dried rapidly and kept in air-tight containers. For tea making, leaves should be dried in early summer (June or July in New England). A decoction of the fresh root is often useful as a treatment for chronic bronchitis but is used more frequently in Europe than in America. The dose is one to two tablespoonsful three times a day and another spoonful at bedtime if needed.

Fresh leaves can be macerated and used as a poultice for external application to help relieve chest congestion.

Angelica stems intended for candying should be collected in midsummer (late July or early August in New England).

Cut stems about four inches long. To candy the stems, cut in four-inch lengths. Boil until tender. Remove from water, peel and then boil again until the stems turn green. Dry and weigh the stems. Measure an equal amount of sugar or honey. Place stems in a shallow earthenware bowl and sprinkle evenly with the sugar or honey. Allow them to remain for twenty-four hours, then put in an enamel pot and boil for ten minutes. Strain juice off and add a little extra sugar or honey (about one-half cup). Boil the juice, partially cool, and put the stems in the thickened juice for a few minutes. Remove stems and put on a plate to dry in a warm place.

Angelica atropurpurea, commonly called masterwort, is found growing wild in moist locations in the United States from the Canadian border as far south as Delaware. It has similar properties and uses to those of *A. archangelica*.

BEE BALM

BEE BALM   *Monarda didyma* L.
("BERGAMOT," "OSWEGO TEA")

LABIATAE

Bee balm is a hardy perennial whose strong, square stems proclaim it to be of the mint family, a fact which its heady fragrance confirms. Bees are attracted to it and in July and August swarm around its scarlet

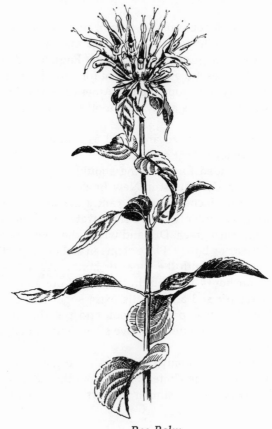

Bee Balm

blossoms, which is the reason for its common name. Hummingbirds select their host flowers by color rather than scent and are constant visitors to the bright red blooms on sunny afternoons.

Bergamot is another common name for *Monarda didyma*, derived from its perfume, which is reminiscent of the "essence of Bergamot" expressed from the fruit rinds of *Citrus bergamia*. This essence is often used as a substitute for oil of Neroli distilled at Grasse from the blossoms of the bitter orange. Both are used in making perfume.

The plant grows to about three feet in good moist garden soil. It is a sparkling decoration to a border or as a background for lower-growing sweet woodruff, melissa, or horehound. Its botanic name honors Dr. Nicolas Monardes, the sixteenth-century Spanish author-physician who wrote *Joyful Newes Out of the New Founde World*. Its third common name, oswego tea, attests to its popularity as a beverage.

The leaves of bee balm grow in pairs, pointed, slightly serrated, and somewhat rough. Large terminal flower whorls are supported by pale-green bracts tinged with red. Both leaves and flowers are carminative and aromatic. Like all the mints, monarda is a pleasant flavored healthy tea for general use. It can also be used medicinally for flatulence, nausea, and/or vomiting.

BORAGE

BORAGE   *Borago officinalis* L.
                                              BORAGINACEAE

Borage, a member of the same family as comfrey (my favorite medicinal herb), shares a few of its virtues and its decorative value to the garden. Unlike comfrey, it is not perennial but self-seeds to such a generous extent that, once a plant is established, it will continue to provide new plants yearly. Plants are about one foot high, with round, rough-textured leaves, alternately placed on the hollow, pithy stem. The flowers are bright blue and star shaped with prominent black anthers forming a central cone.

Borage leaves have a cucumber-like fragrance, and like the cucumber, impart a nice coolness to salads or summer drinks.

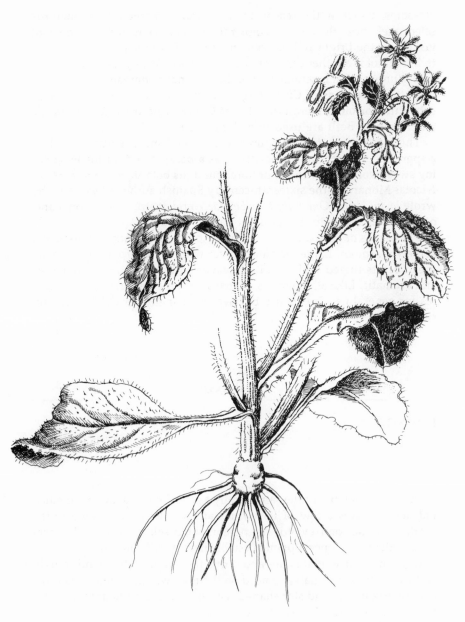

Borage

Like comfrey, the whole plant contains potassium and calcium, combined with mineral acids. Diuretic, demulcent, emollient, it is a popular herbal remedy for fevers, chest complaints, and skin blemishes. Due to the saline mucilage of stems and leaves, it helps the kidneys to carry off feverish catarrhs.

The flowers, candied, are a decoration to any dessert—sherbet or cake—or as a candy. The fresh blue blossoms are a pleasant addition to a punch bowl.

Borage is a perfect example of companionable planting—systematic placing of plants which protect or stimulate another plant next to it in the garden. Borage is the helpmate of the strawberry plant, keeping it free of disease or marauding insects. In my garden it has very amiably self-seeded around the strawberry bed each year.

BUGLE

BUGLE
Ajuga reptans L.
LABIATAE

The low-growing perennial bugle is under the beneficent influence of Venus. The purple lower leaves are oblong, obtuse with gently toothed edges, and from this creeping mass of color six- to eight-inch stalks flower in early summer. Purple-blue blossoms grow around a spike in whorls, usually about six flowers to the whorl, and in between them are small leaves the same color as the flower which give the entire plant a bluish tone. In late summer, the purple leaves change color and are dark green, splotched with a dull violet. Another variety has green leaves and rose-colored blossoms.

Roots from the reclining stems form new plants every spring, so it is easy to establish a border of *Ajuga*.

The whole plant is used medicinally. It should be gathered for drying when the leaves are at their best and the flowers have just formed—the end of June in Vermont. It is bitter, astringent, aromatic, gently laxative, and sedative.

Herbalists use bugle for coughs, nervousness, and headache, to lower

113

the pulse rate and induce calm, for which purposes an infusion is used, taken internally.

Externally, an infusion can be used as a wet dressing, or the herb can be pounded and made into a poultice with slippery elm and cider vinegar. Either of these methods will be effective for cuts, sores, abrasions, or swollen joints. The leaves and flowers, fresh or dried, put into hot bath water, will restore aching muscles and frayed nerves.

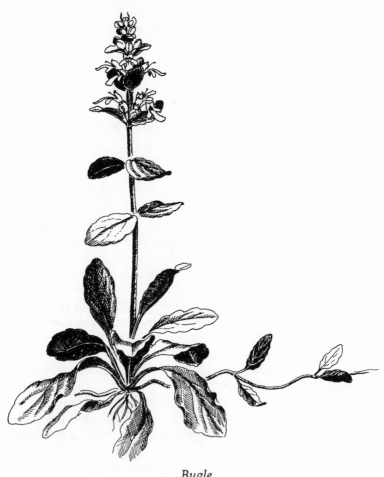

Bugle

CARAWAY

CARAWAY   *Carum carvi* L.
                                                      UMBELLIFERAE

A biennial, caraway grows to two feet high with finely cut leaves and umbels of small white to faintly violet tinted flowers. It was used in ancient times by the Arabs, who brought it into Spain. The seeds were

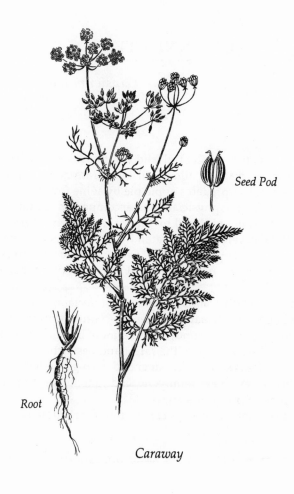

Seed Pod

Root

Caraway

used then, as now, in bread and cakes. Oil from the seeds is used in making Kummel and other alcoholic beverages.

Some curious beliefs were held about caraway in early times. It was said to keep hens and pigeons from straying, and was used in love potions to insure fidelity.

The seeds and oil of caraway are aromatic, stimulant and carminative. They contain a volatile oil, with carvone, which is a hydrocarbon.

The plant seems to adapt to many parts of the world and to a wide variety of soils and climates. In the United States it is often found growing wild, along country roads and in waste places.

CAYENNE PEPPER

CAYENNE   *Capsicum frutescens* L.
                                              SOLANACEAE

Cayenne is a native of Central and South America, but it can be grown as a garden plant in almost all temperate zones, even in Vermont. Its Americanism predates apple pie by some four hundred years. It was mentioned by the physician who accompanied Columbus on his second voyage to America. Used by the mayas of Central America and the Incas of Peru, cayenne is still eaten by the Indians of Mexico as an internal disinfectant. It protects them from amoebic dysentery, which affects visitors from the north who will not use hot pepper on their food.

Cayenne is carminative, antispasmodic, disinfectant, tonic, and stimulant. Samuel Thomson, the early nineteenth-century doctor who started botanic treatment and who founded the Vermont Botanic Medical School in 1836, called *Capsicum* "one of the safest and best articles ever discovered to remove disease." He recommended taking one-half to one teaspoonful in hot water. Every family, he said "should keep on hand two ounces of cayenne for a year's supply."[1]

In herbal treatment today, *Capsicum* is used for rheumatism, arthritis,

---

[1] Samuel Thomson, *Thomsonian Materia Medica.* Albany, N.Y.; 1841, 1847.

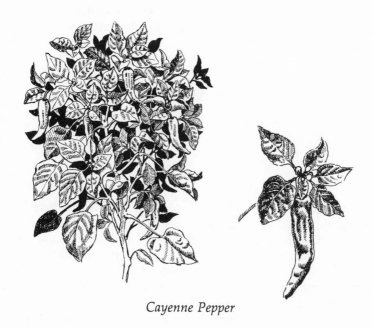

Cayenne Pepper

and as an internal disinfectant and a heart stimulant. A poultice for arthritis and rheumatism is made with:

one part cayenne pepper
equal parts mullein leaves and slippery elm powder
cider vinegar to dampen the mixture

Many familiar soft drinks, ginger ale and cream soda for example, contain *Capsicum* along with other aboriginal botanicals such as vanilla, ginger, allspice, and sarsaparilla.

Cayenne used as a fumigant is safe and efficient in ridding buildings of vermin. Put a heaping tablespoon of the dried and powdered pepper in a shallow pan over a low flame and allow the fumes to pervade the air. Mice, rats, even cockroaches abhor the fumes, which are quite harmless to humans and domestic pets.

A container of red pepper or a small bottle of pepper sauce (cayenne in vinegar) is a sensible protection to carry when you travel in countries where the preparation and serving of food is not always sanitary. Because it is known throughout the world as a condiment, you can sprinkle cayenne on your food without appearing rude or tactless.

CELANDINE

CELANDINE   *Chelidonium majus* L.
                                                PAPAVERACEAE

The greater celandine, under the protection of the Sun, is found growing along old stone walls and the foundations of barns. Look for it on the periphery of human habitation. It is a reliable perennial, usually found in the same place year after year. The stem is round and slender, and when broken, exudes an orange-colored juice which is of medicinal value in curing simple warts. The leaves are light green, about eight inches long, divided to the midriff in wavy rounded sections. The flowers grow in loose, terminal umbels, have four yellow petals, and bloom throughout the summer months. They are followed by long, thin, seed pods in autumn. Pliny wrote that its name, *Chelidonium*, was derived from the Greek word for the swallow, "chelidon," because the blossoming of the plant coincided with the arrival of the swallows in summer, and it faded when they migrated in the fall. Pliny said that the juice of celandine was used by the swallows to give sight to their young. This juice is used by herbalists today to remove film from the eyes. Gerard described the juice as being "good to sharpen sight . . . especially being boiled with honey in a brassen vessel, as Dioscorides teacheth."

I would disagree with the boiling as it would destroy the therapeutic value of the honey if not the celandine. I might add that natural honey, unboiled, as it comes from the comb, has been used successfully to cure cataracts on the eye in one case that I know.

I have good results in curing sties by touching them with the raw juice of the stem, one or two applications being all that was necessary.

Celandine contains at least twenty-five alkaloids, including chelidonine and cherlerythrine, the latter narcotic and poisonous.

The leaves and stems, steeped in warm milk, are a safe and effective eye-wash. The fresh orange-colored juice of the stems should be rubbed directly on warts, corns, and calluses, taking care not to let the juice stand on any other parts of the skin. This treatment should be repeated two or three times a day.

A fomentation is said to be good for the relief of toothache, but this is one use of celandine that I have not tried. It is used in parts of England, notably Sussex.

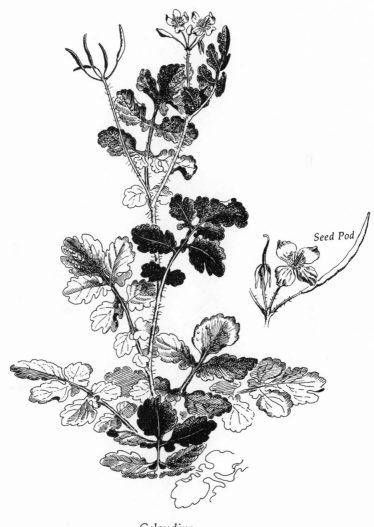

Seed Pod

Celandine

CLOVER

RED CLOVER
("FIELD CLOVER")

Trifolium pratense L.

LEGUMINOSAE

Trifolium pratense, naturalized from Europe, grows best in light, sandy soil, in fields and meadows. The leaves, as its name indicates (*Trifolium*),

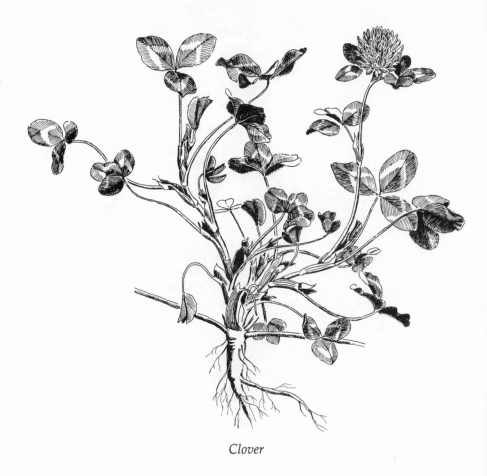

Clover

are divided into three leaflets. The flower heads are egg-shaped, about one inch long with red to purplish flowers.

Medically, red clover is alterative, diuretic, and sedative. Taken over a long period of time, an infusion of red clover acts as a stimulant to the liver and bladder. Poultices and fomentations have been used as a traditional local treatment for cancerous growths. Medical testing at the present time is exploring the use of the plant as a cancer deterrent.

The flowers are the part used. Dried or fresh they combine well with many other herbs to make a palatable and healthy tea; the nectar at the base of the florets retains its saccharine secretion giving a natural sweetness to the infusion.

CORIANDER

CORIANDER   *Coriandrum sativum* L.
                           UMBRELLIFERAE

Coriander is a handsome annual growing one to three feet high. The lower leaves are irregularly cut, like those of parsley. The upper leaves are thin, linear, and resemble dill, but are somewhat shorter and coarser.

Coriander seeds are used in pickles and curry powder. In Mexico the leaves are called *cilantro*, are sold in every market, and are a favorite herb to cook with black beans, a staple food south of the border.

Medicinally coriander is a stimulant, aromatic and carminative. It contains a volatile oil and the fruit (or seed) contains malic acid, tannin, ash and some fatty matter.

Coriander is an herb from the East; always popular in Egypt, it is still used for flavoring there to such an extent that local dishes are sometimes a bit too much for Western palates. The Romans brought coriander to England, and from there the early colonists ordered the seeds for their gardens in the New World.

121

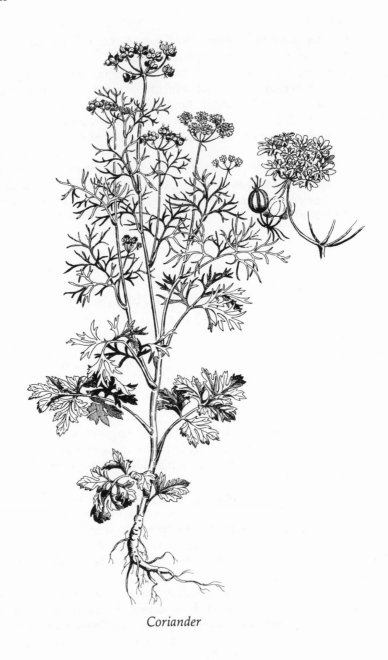

Coriander

COUCH GRASS

COUCH GRASS   *Agropyron repens* (L.) Beauv.
("WITCH," "DOG," "QUACK,"
OR "TWITCH GRASS")

GRAMINEAE

The botanical name of this omnipresent grass comes from two Greek words; *agros* (field) and *puros* (wheat). The number of common names by which it is known gives evidence to widespread use and abuse by man and man's best friend, the dog. Dogs and cats seek it out when they are sick, and cure themselves.

Agropyron repens was well known to Dioscorides, who found it useful for stones in the bladder, taken as a decoction. Dodoen's *A Niewe Herball* shows a wood engraving of the plant, and it was well thought of by Gerard, who felt that, although it was "an unwelcome guest to fields and gardens," its virtues as a medicine "do recompense those hurts." He thought it useful to "openeth the stoppings of the liver." Culpepper praised it for "virtues in treating kidney diseases."

A description of couch grass is quite unnecessary: Those who live in the country know it all too well; those who live in the city can order the dried rhizomes, the part used medicinally, from a supplier of botanicals. (See Appendix IV for list of suppliers.)

The rhizome is diuretic, demulcent, emollient, and tonic. It contains triticum (a carbohydrate somewhat like inulin), sugar, inosite, mucilage, and acid malates.

It is used for bladder, liver, and gall-bladder troubles, and irritations of the urinary tract.

In France, it has been, and still is in country districts, considered an excellent spring tonic. It is taken as a tisane, or tea.

For use as an infusion take according to directions for standard brew. Take up to two cupfuls a day, a gulp at a time. A decoction may be used as a tonic, taken cold, one-half to one cup a day. (See directions for decoction in Chapter IV.)

I discovered an interesting use for quack grass fifteen years ago

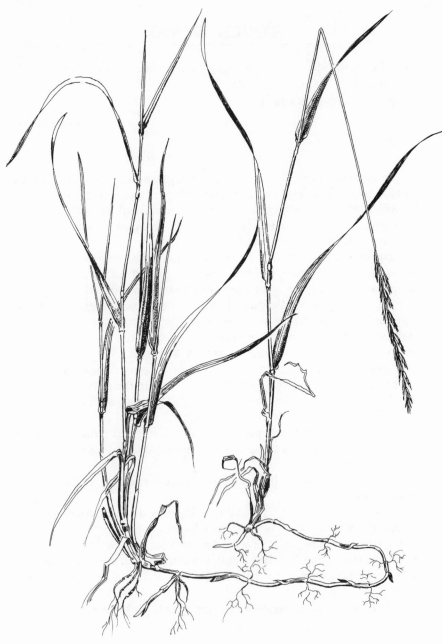

Couch Grass

when I began to prepare a garden plot where the soil had not been under cultivation for sixty years. It was a mass of quack grass. A neighbor rototilled the plot. I shook all the soil from the roots and covered it with as much organic kitchen waste as my household and friends could supply, then replaced the quack grass roots on top of this and covered it with wood ashes. This was in October. By the next June, I planted my first garden in the new location. It grew abundantly.

DILL

DILL   *Anethum graveolens* L.
UMBELLIFERAE

The feathery leaves of dill topped by corymbs of yellow flowers which form seeds in July or August are a familiar sight in almost every garden. Dill seeds, and fresh dill weed, are a deservedly popular and easily recognized flavor in pickles and sauces for fish. They add zest to salads, mayonnaise and all bland vegetables.

The name dill is believed to be derived from an old Norse word, *dilla*, meaning to lull, and descriptive of the herb's ability to relieve pains from gas in the stomach.

Dill is an annual plant which grows to two and one-half feet on a single, smooth stalk. An oil of dill containing limonene and carvone is contained in the seeds. Its medical properties are stimulant, carminative and aromatic.

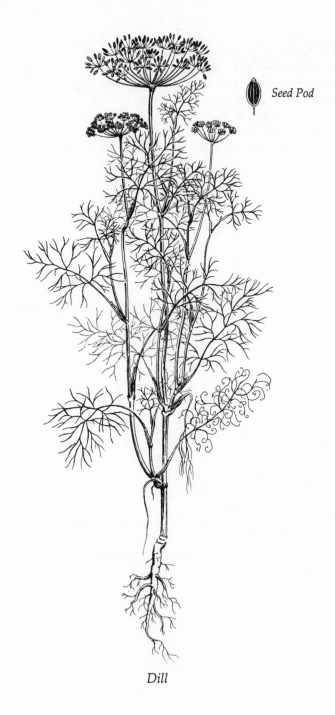

Seed Pod

Dill

ELDER

COMMON ELDER
("SWEET," "COMMON," OR
"BLACK ELDER")

Sambucus canadensis L.[1]

CAPRIFOLIACEAE

American elder grows four to ten feet high. The leaves are composed of five to seven leaflets, oval with sharply acute tips and serrated edges. White flowers grow on flat terminal cymes. The berries turn from green to light red to dark red and purple-black when ripe.

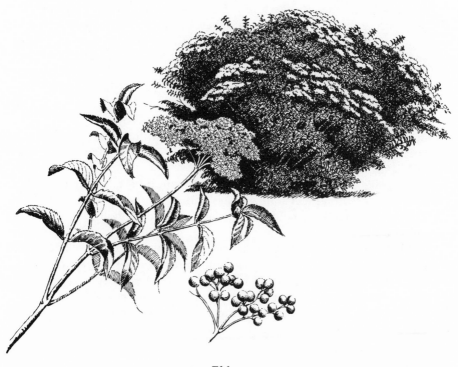

Elder

[1] *S. canadensis* is an American species related to the European *S. nigra*.

Bark constituents: viburnic acid; a soft resin; traces of a volatile oil; tannic acid; chlorophyll; grape sugar; gum; starch; pectin; fat; wax; alkaline; and earthy salts.

Bark medicinal action: purgative, emetic, diuretic.

Leaf constituents: an alkaloid, sambucine, a purgative resin; and a glycocide, sambunirin. When fresh, the leaves contain a trace (about 0.16 percent) hydrocyanic acid, cane sugar, invertin, potassium nitrate, and eldrin, a crystalline substance.

Leaves are used in an ointment that is a domestic remedy for bruises, sprains, chilblains, and hard-to-cure skin irritations. In the sixteenth and seventeenth centuries it was believed that the leaves of the elder should be gathered on the last day of April, and hung on doors and windows to prevent witches from entering the house.

A salve useful in treating swellings, piles (hemorrhoids), and tumors is made from a handful each of elder leaves, comfrey leaves, plantain, mugwort, ground ivy, and thyme leaves. Chop finely, barely cover with water, bring to a boil, then simmer for thirty minutes. Strain. Add an equal amount of olive or safflower oil and simmer until all the water has evaporated. Add enough beeswax to make a soft salve consistency.

The elder flower contains a semi-solid volatile oil (about 0.32 percent), which, when the leaves dry, decreases.

The flowers, fresh or dry, are used to make infusions. A tea is useful in treating bronchitis and bringing out the rash in measles and other eruptive diseases. Used as a skin lotion, it is a gentle stimulant and a mild astringent.

To make elderberry water for a skin lotion, fill a quart jar with the blossoms, pour on them boiling water until the jar is three-quarters full. Cool, add enough alcohol to fill the jar, let stand six hours, strain, and bottle for use.

Elderberry flower and peppermint tea, if taken every few hours in the very first stages of influenza, will ward off a serious attack. It is diaphoretic; so stay in bed and keep well covered as perspiration starts. It is also a very mild laxative, which will keep the system clear.

For inflammation of the bladder and the mucous lining of the urinary passage, mix together thoroughly equal parts of:

elderberry flowers
St. John's-wort (whole herb)
chamomile flowers
corn silk
blackberry leaves

Use from two to three teaspoonfuls to a cup of boiling water. Let stand until cold. Strain. Take one cup three times a day, before meals.

To remove freckles, soak flowers in water overnight, strain and use as a wash several times a day.

The elder was known to the Egyptians, listed by Hippocrates in his *materia medica*, and mentioned by Pliny, Culpepper, John Evelyn, and Father Sebastian Kneipp as a blood purifier. For this purpose a tea should be taken, one cup a day, before breakfast, for one week.

The dried berries are a cure for diarrhea.

Doctors in Europe prescribe pure elderberry juice, taken daily for five days or more, for trigeminal neuralgia and sciatica.

Like many other plants which have been used and loved over the centuries, elder has given rise to folklore. It was believed that it could not be struck by lightning and for that reason should be planted near the house. It was also thought to protect those in the house from disease and evil spirits. A twig, carried close to the body, was thought to be a charm to give health and good luck.

Elderberry Wine

Gather the ripe berries on a dry day, separate them from the stems and put in an earthenware crock. Cover with boiling water to the amount of one gallon of water to every two gallons of berries. Press berries into the water with a wooden spoon or potato masher. Cover and let stand twenty-four hours. Strain through a sieve, mashing out all possible juice. Measure the juice and add three pounds of sugar (or honey) to each gallon of juice. Toss in a small handful of cloves and a little grated fresh ginger. Pour back into the crock and add one package dry yeast dissolved in one-quarter cup of the juice. Cover, let stand until it stops working (bubbling). Strain through cheesecloth and bottle in gallon jugs. After two months decant into wine bottles and cork tightly.

Elderberry Flower Wine

Put one quart of fresh flowers in an earthenware crock. Pour over them three gallons boiling water in which nine pounds of sugar (or seven pounds of honey) have been dissolved. Allow to cool. Add juice of one lemon, three pounds of raisins, and one package of dry yeast dissolved in one-quarter cup of lukewarm juice. Let stand in a crock until it stops working (about ten days). Strain through cheesecloth and bottle in gallon jug. After three months decant into wine bottles and cork tightly.

Elderberry Jelly

Cook ripe berries and strain through jelly bag. Cook tart crab apples, mash and strain through jelly bag. Combine one-half cup of crab apple juice to each cup elderberry juice. Add three-quarters cup of sugar, or honey, to each cup of juice. Bring to brisk boil and then boil gently until the amount that will stick to the spoon thickens when it cools. Have sterilized jars ready and pour the jelly. Wait ten minutes and pour melted paraffin on top.

EVENING PRIMROSE

EVENING PRIMROSE   *Oenothera biennis* L.
                                           ONAGRACEAE

Evening primrose is native to the United States. A biennial, it is found along roadsides and in dry meadows. The long lanceolate leaves, three to five inches with a width of one or two inches, are pointed and entire. The main stem has terminal yellow flowers.

Medicinally, evening primrose is astringent, mucilaginous, sedative. The whole herb is used. It is useful in gastrointestinal and hepatic ailments, useful for coughs and mental depression.

It is used in salve form, combined with other herbs, for skin irritations.

For use as infusion make a standard brew; use one cup a day, taking one mouthful at a time.

Tincture: Five to forty drops as needed in a half-cup of water.

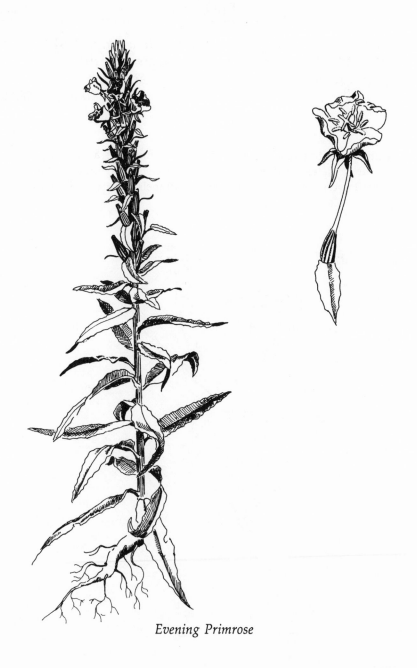

Evening Primrose

FENNEL

FENNEL	*Foeniculum vulgare* Mill.
FLORENCE FENNEL	*F. vulgare* var. dulce
("FINNOCHIO")	Batt. and Trab.
	UMBELLIFERAE

Fennel is native to Europe but is usually found as a garden plant in the United States. It is a feathery-leaved perennial or biannual with yellow flowers appearing on terminal umbels. It grows best in soils

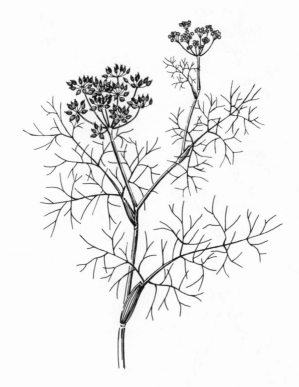

Fennel

with a lime content. All parts of the plant are used—root, herb, and seeds. Pliny gave twenty-two uses for fennel, and Gerard said, "of fennel, roses, vervain, rue, and celandine, is made a water good to cleare the sight of eine."

The Romans cultivated fennel for its aromatic seeds and edible roots. Ancient herbalists believed that fennel had a very beneficial effect on the eyesight and, in Italy, oily fish cooked with it was thought to be easier to digest. Another widely held belief was that drinking fennel tea or broth would have a slimming effect on those who were overweight. This may have originated with the Greeks whose name for it, "marathon," was derived from the verb "maraino," to grow thin.

Fennel's principal constituents are anethole and fenchone, both found in the volatile oil. It is antispasmodic, aromatic, carminative, diuretic, galactagogue (milk forming), stimulant, and stomachic.

Fennel is useful to relieve abdominal cramps and flatulence, and to get rid of mucus. It stimulates the formation and flow of milk in nursing mothers if taken as a decoction of the seed in barley water. A decoction of the seed, strained and diluted with an equal part of water, is a home remedy for eyestrain or to wash a foreign substance from the eye.

Oil of fennel eases muscular or rheumatic pains.

Florence fennel, like the common fennel, grows best in somewhat limey soil, but it needs a richer earth. The root is bulbous and larger, but the plant does not grow as tall. It is best to find a spot in the garden away from other herbs, particularly basil, as both fennels have an adverse effect on other plants.

FEVERFEW

FEVERFEW   *Tanacetum parthenium* (L.) Schultz Bip.
                 (*Chrysanthemum parthenium* Bernh.)
                                              COMPOSITAE

The name feverfew is a corruption of "febrifuge," a word meaning to allay fever, which describes this herb nicely. It is carminative, aperient, and a mild nervine with a bitter taste.

133

Feverfew is small, about two feet high, with alternate leaves, cut deeply and irregularly like other chrysanthemums. The flowers are similar to chamomile with white florets, but the yellow centers are flat rather than conical. In some species the entire flower is yellow.

Early spring is the best time to plant feverfew. Choose a rich, loamy soil in full sun. Once the plants are established, they can be divided to make two or three new plants. Cuttings can be taken from young basal shoots, which should be cut back to three inches when they are set in the soil. Seeds may be started indoors to be put in a sunny location in May or June.

Feverfew gives protection from the bites and stings of mosquitoes,

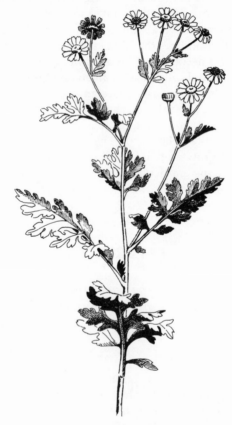

Feverfew

bees, flies, and gnats. Use a double strength standard brew to bathe hands, arms, face, and legs. Allow it to dry on the skin. Applications may be made every few hours. Because feverfew is a relative of pyrethrum, a potent insecticide, it is not surprising that it, too, is distasteful to insects.

Culpepper says of feverfew, "Venus commands this herb, and has commended it to succor her sisters [women], to be a general strengthener of their wombs, and to remedy such infirmities as a careless midwife has there caused." I have no personal experience with feverfew for the "infirmities" related by Culpepper, but as he had a large practice in Red Lion Street dating from the 1640's and was himself the father of seven children, I see no reason to doubt him.

When I recommend feverfew tea (standard brew) for headache and low fever, I am on firm and familiar ground. It has a mild tranquilizing effect and is especially good for headaches caused by tension or fatigue. The same infusion may be taken, cold, as a tonic. The dose for this use is one-half to one teaspoonful at a time, taken between meals.

GARLIC

GARLIC   *Allium sativum* L.
                                        LILIACEAE

This powerful herb, ruled by Mars, has been known and valued for more than five thousand years. In ancient Egypt fifteen pounds of garlic would buy one able-bodied slave. Wild garlic, *Allium reticulatum,* is thought to be the famous "Moly" of Homer. Hermes gave it to Ulysses, who used it to subdue Circe, thus rescuing his sailors whom she had turned into swine.

The Roman legions were given survival rations of caraway bread and garlic when they were fighting away from home. When Sir John Harington composed his poetic version of the cures used at the medical School of Salerno in 1607, garlic received top priority as a disinfectant:

> *Six things that are here in order shall ensue,*
> *Against all poysens have a secret power,*

> *Peare, Garlicke, Reddish Roots, Rape and Rue*
> *But Garlicke chief, for they that it devoure,*
> *May drink and care not who their drink do brew,*
> *May walke in aires infected every houre.*

Maximilian, Prince of Weid, was cured from what was considered a hopeless case of scurvy at Fort Clark in 1834, when some Indian children gathered wild garlic which was administered to him by a Negro

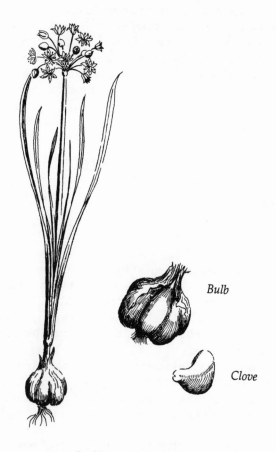

Bulb

Clove

Garlic

cook. The writings of early white frontier doctors tell us that the Winnebagos and Dakotas used garlic to relieve wasp and bee stings. Garlic even inspired some place names in the United States. Chicago, in the language of the Algonquin-speaking Indians of northeastern Illinois, meant "place of the wild garlic."

A nineteenth-century medical book, *The Family Doctor*, published in 1869, lists garlic as "stimulant, diuretic, expectorant, deobstructant," and recommends its use in chronic catarrhs, humoral asthma, worms, epilepsy, and dropsy.

We know today that garlic is also alterative, antiseptic, diaphoretic, antispasmodic, vulnerary, antibiotic. It has up to 0.9 percent of volatile oil containing diallyl disulphide and allylpropyl disulphide, and glucoside, allin, which is hydrolyzed by the enzyme, allisin, to form volatile oil and fructose.

Pliny listed more than sixty diseases for which garlic was a cure. It is well known today that garlic is effective against both "staph" and "strep" infections and is effective in treatment of typhoid, enteritis, and cholera. High in sulphur, garlic is effective in treatment of internal and external infections. It acts by combining with harmful bacteria to stop their action, allowing healthful bacteria to grow back. It cures open wounds through the regeneration of epidermal cells. It is a specific for bronchitis, asthma, high blood pressure, stomach ulcers, chronic colitis, all respiratory infections, colds, influenza, urinary tract infections, and cardiovascular problems. As a preventive medicine, it has no equal in the home.

At the faintest sign of sore throat, running nose, or aching bones, simply take a clove of fresh garlic, peel, cut in half, and place one-half in each cheek, allowing the juice to be absorbed in the saliva and pervade the system. The odor can be masked by use of anise, cinnamon, or caraway seeds. Both garlic tablets and capsules are available for those who cannot adjust to the garlic odor.

The following five methods of preparing garlic for home use are easy and effective.

Oil of Garlic

ια.

Peel and mince eight ounces of garlic. Put in a jar and cover with warm olive oil. Turn the jar several times a day for four days, strain the juice, put it back in the jar, and keep in a cool place. For internal use, the dose can be from ten drops to one teaspoonful three or four times a day.

Garlic Cough Medicine

Place one pound of peeled and sliced garlic in a jar and cover with a mixture of equal parts of apple-cider vinegar and water. Let stand for four or five hours, strain, and add an equal amount of honey. Keep the juice in a cool place and shake well before using. One tablespoonful may be taken three or four times a day.

For bronchitis put two whole, peeled cloves of garlic through a press, add to one cup of honey, and take the entire cupful, a spoonful at a time, during a twenty-four hour period.

Fresh-grated garlic or expressed juice may be put directly on any external wound or infection.

In using garlic as a healthy item of diet, remember that boiling destroys the medicinal properties. Always add it to soups, stews, vegetables, just before serving. Garlic bread has always been considered a gourmet addition to the serving of a crisp green salad or home-made soup.

An example of the immunity to disease that garlic gives was the famous Four Thieves Vinegar. During the plague of 1722, in the city of Marseilles, four thieves achieved immunity through daily doses of garlic vinegar, which allowed them to plunder the dead bodies of plague victims without contracting the disease.

No household should ever be without a good supply of fresh garlic. If you have even a small garden, garlic is easy to grow and harvest. Divide the bulb into its separate cloves and plant in the fall in well-tilled, rich, loamy soil, well drained. It will be ready to harvest the following summer.

In World War I the army discovered the efficacy of garlic as a disinfectant for wounds, and it was credited with saving many lives. It is high in organic sulphur, vitamins, and minerals. For those involved in the pressures and anxieties of economic survival, it is comforting to know that the readily available and inexpensive garlic helps to lower hypertension, equalizes blood circulation, and is active against tumor formation. It is useful in such diverse conditions as athlete's foot, diabetes, rheumatism, sciatica, and pimples.

GROUND-IVY

GROUND-IVY
("GILL-OVER-THE-HILL,"
"ALE-HOOF")

Glechoma hederacea L.

LABIATAE

This little herb belongs to Venus, the planet who rules ease, comfort, and love; it is never very far from human habitation, seemingly waiting, inconspicuous, until it is needed. It is tonic, astringent, diuretic, antiscorbutic, and mildly stimulant. It can be used as a home remedy for digestive and kidney diseases.

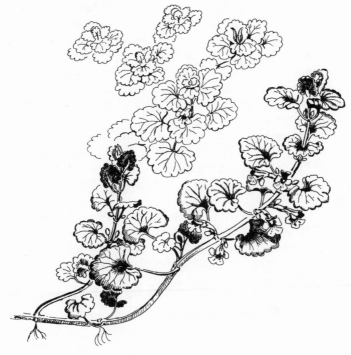

Ground Ivy

Dioscorides said that "half a dram of the leaves being drunk in foure ounces and a half of faire water for forty or fifty days together is a remedy against sciatica or ache in the hucklebone." This might be efficacious in chronic sciatica; I have only treated sporadic, acute cases, usually when they occurred as an occupational disease. For such cases other herbs are stronger and more direct.

Culpepper calls ground-ivy "a singular herb for all inward wounds." He says "the juice, dropped into the ear doth wonderfully help the noise and singing in them, and helpeth the hearing which is decayed."

Gerard recommended a combination of ground-ivy, celandine, and English daisies in equal parts, bruised and strained, put into rose water with a little sugar and "dropped with a feather into the eies" which, he said, "taketh away all manner of inflammation, spots, webs, itch, smarting, or any grief whatsoever in the eyes. . . ." He also gave a description of the plant in the original publication of *The Herball or General Historie of Plantes* (1597) which cannot be improved on; so I will quote it here:

"Ground ivy is a low or base herbe, it creepeth and spread upon the ground hither and thither all about, with many stalks of uncertain length, slender, and like those of the vine: thereupon grow leaves something broad and round: amongst which come forth the floures gaping like little hoods, not unlike those of Germander, of a purplish blew colour; the whole plant is of a strong smell and bitter taste." It grew then, as now, in "tilled and in untilled places . . . upon banks under hedges, and by the sides of houses."

On the southeast side of my house, ground-ivy grows just as Gerard said, on a bank shaded by an elderberry hedge. The whole herb is used medicinally. I have had good results from an infusion, taken internally, to relieve upset stomach and headache caused by digestive disturbance and to reduce low fever.

For an eye-wash, I have infused two parts gill-over-the-hill with one part celandine, added a little honey, and obtained immediate relief. Gerard's addition of English daisies would be good, I am sure, but I have not found it necessary, and I have a limited supply, whose pink and white gaiety I enjoy too much to cut. I disagree with Gerard's use of sugar. Honey is preferable because of its ability to absorb oxygen, without which a film over the eye cannot exist.

HAWKWEED

HAWKWEED   *Hieracium pilosella* L.
                                COMPOSITAE

There are at least seven hundred species of *Hieracium,* mostly in the north temperate zone and the Andes of South America.

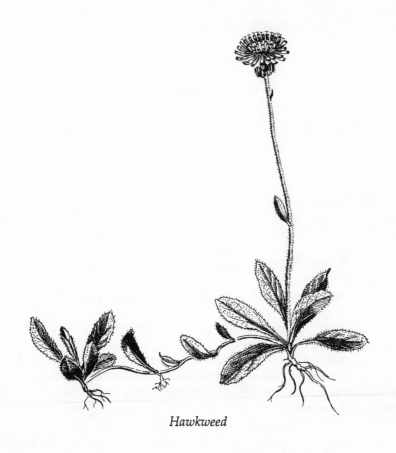

Hawkweed

Hawkweed, sometimes called mouse-ear hawkweed, is astringent, chologogic, and diuretic. It checks diarrhea and is a soothing gargle for mild sore throat. For both purposes it is used in the form of an infusion, standard brew.

Hawkweed is a perennial wildflower usually found in dry soil. Spatulate leaves form a basal rosette from which orange or yellow flowers, similar to the dandelion, grow on bare stems about three to five inches high. Country and suburban dwellers know that it can be seen all summer, growing in small patches at the edge of lawns, gardens, fields, and roads. It is a useful remedy for vacationers in the country to know and look for, as it is a mild and safe treatment for two common complaints due to change of diet and climate—sore throat and diarrhea.

HOREHOUND

HOREHOUND   *Marrubium vulgare* L.
                                                    LABIATAE

A low, about six to eight inches, perennial with cordate–ovate, downy leaves and small white flowers growing in axillary whorls, horehound is a decorative and useful plant which should be included in every herb garden.

The botanical name, *Marrubium,* is derived from the Hebrew word marrob, or "bitter juice."

Medicinally horehound is a bitter tonic, an expectorant, a decongestant, and a diuretic.

Horehound contains a bitter principle, marubium; resin; tannin; a volatile oil; sugar and wax.

Folk medicine has always relied on horehound to cure bronchitis, coughs, and chronic catarrh. Herbalists recommend it for increasing the circulation, and to aid in liver trouble and painful menstruation. For all the above complaints a standard brew may be sweetened with honey and taken, two tablespoonsful at a time, three or four times a day.

A horehound cough syrup can be made by stirring a strong infusion into a cup of honey to which one tablespoon of lemon juice has been added.

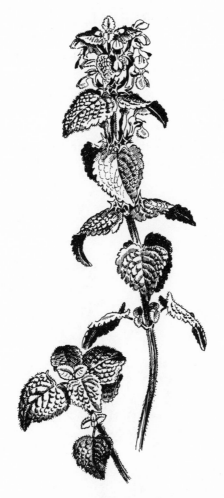

Horehound

Horehound candy is easy to make and keeps well in jars or wrapped in wax paper. To one cup of honey add one cup brown sugar and one tablespoon butter. Stir an infusion made from one handful of the whole, fresh plant into one-half cup boiling water. Cook until a few drops will form a soft ball when dropped in a cup of cold water. Pour on a buttered plate, score while warm, cut when cold.

143

HORSETAIL

HORSETAIL   *Equisetum arvense* L.
  ("SHAVEGRASS," "PEWTERWURT,"
  "BOTTLEBRUSH")

EQUISETACEAE

The young stems of horsetail that appear in spring are bare of leaves and resemble a slim asparagus, attaining a height of eight or ten inches.

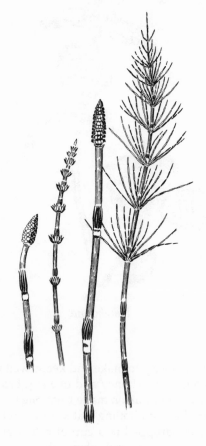

Horsetail

These die down and in July are followed by what Culpepper aptly describes as "hard, rough, hollow stalks, joined at sundry places at the top, a foot high, so made as if the lower parts were put into the upper, where grow on each side a bush of small long rush-like hard leaves, each part ressembling a horsetail."

The *Equisetum* we see today growing in damp areas are the minuscule descendants of twenty- to thirty-foot trees which flourished in the Carboniferous age, 300 million years ago. Fossil impressions, called "Calamites," often appear on the surface of coal.

The stems, the part we use medicinally, can be fresh or dried. They are diuretic, astringent, hemostatic, and vulnerary.

An infusion made by steeping two teaspoonsful of *Equisetum* stems in one cup of boiling water may be taken, one cup a day, for urinary infections. This infusion may also be used as a gargle for sore gums, or as a wash for skin eruptions.

A decoction, thickened with flour, slippery elm, or beaten egg white is useful as a poultice for ruptures, wounds, or arthritic pains.

HYSSOP

HYSSOP	*Hyssopus officinalis* L.
	LABIATAE

This hardy, perennial herb is ruled by Jupiter. A neat, bushy plant, it grows to two feet high. The stem is square, and the narrow leaves resemble tarragon. There are several varieties, each bearing a different color flower—white, pink, and lavender. It can be started from seeds, cuttings, or root division. It thrives best in a light, somewhat sandy soil.

The leaves and flowers are expectorant, diaphoretic, stimulant, pectoral, and carminative. The plant contains a volatile oil, which is the source of hyssop's diaphoretic qualities.

Gerard quotes Dioscorides as saying that hyssop boiled with rue and honey helps those that have coughs, shortness of breath, and wheezing. He recommends "The green herb, bruised with a little sugar put thereto," to heal any "cut or green wound." We would amend his formula to use honey instead of sugar.

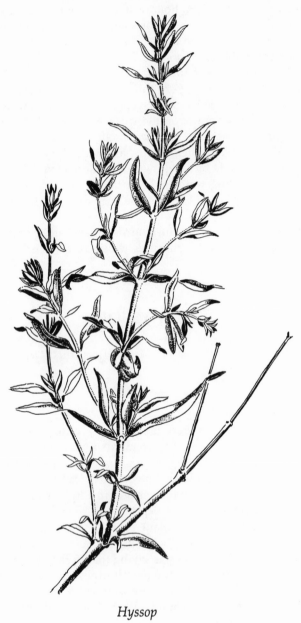

Hyssop

Given warm as an infusion, hyssop works well to break up chronic catarrh and may safely be taken as often as needed. For this purpose horehound and pennyroyal may be added to the infusion.

Locally applied, an infusion will take away discoloration from bruises. Country housewives in the nineteenth century used a decoction of tops and flowers for a treatment for rheumatism. It works. I add a teaspoon of natural (unboiled) honey and one of cider vinegar (without preservatives) to each pint of the decoction.

Hyssop is an important ingredient in the liqueur Chartreuse and can be used to make a delicious home cordial. (See directions under Lemon Balm, Chapter VII.)

Like the mints, hyssop was a favorite "strewing herb" in seventeenth-century England.

All of the above uses of hyssop are reliable, but there are other herbs, just as available, that have the same medicinal qualities. My greatest use for hyssop is as a pleasant-smelling, inexpensive, non-toxic cleaning agent for floors, bathroom fixtures, flower pots, and linens.

The name "hyssop" came from the Greek "azob," a holy herb, because of its use in cleaning sacred places. I make a double strength infusion (double standard brew), strain it, and add to a pail of warm water. If you have cats or dogs, pennyroyal may be added to the infusion as an insurance against fleas hiding in any crevices of floor or wall.

A strained, strong infusion of hyssop can be poured into the washing machine during the rinse cycle to give linens a gentle bleach.

LADY'S MANTLE

LADY'S MANTLE   *Alchemilla xanthochlora* Rothm.
                     (*Alchemilla vulgaris* auct.)
                                        ROSACEAE

Venus is the patron planet of this eighteen-inch high plant, whose large, rounded leaves are palmate, seven- to nine-lobed, evenly and finely toothed. Tiny, yellow-green, star-shaped flowers form loose panicles. Its botanic name, *Alchemilla,* comes from the Arabic word for

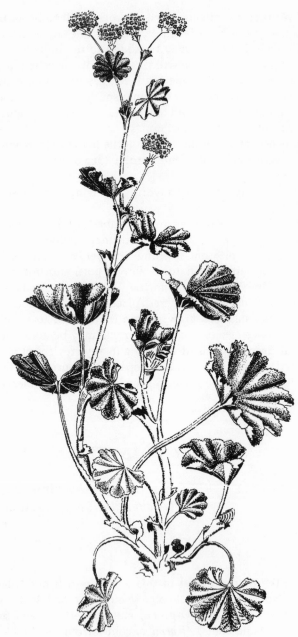

Lady's Mantle

alchemist, "alkemelych," the scientists who predated our modern chemists. The name gives us yet another reminder that the plants that serve us well today were known and used in all ages.

It is said that the diamond-like drops of dew, which gather in the accordion-pleated leaves of *Alchemilla,* were thought by the alchemists to undergo some subtly benign influence from the plant and were used in many mystic potions.

In 1532 Tragus (Jerome Bock) first called the plant Lady's Mantle or "Frauenmantle" (in German), when he published his *History of Plants,* a name which Linnaeus adopted in his classification.

The whole herb is used, as well as the root, for both internal and external treatment. The plant should be gathered for drying when in full bloom, but the root may be used fresh as well as dry. It can be found growing wild in shaded woodlands or can be grown easily from seed in our gardens, where it forms an unusual accent plant. In cultivation it will tolerate sunny locations as well as shade.

Lady's Mantle is astringent, styptic, tonic, and vulnerary. Culpepper says that "It is proper for those wounds that have inflammation, and is effective to stay bleedings, vomitings, and fluxes of all sorts; . . ."

An infusion taken internally is good for loss of appetite, rheumatism, stomach trouble, diarrhea, and excessive menstruation, and as a blood coagulant. It makes an excellent mouthwash and is effective to stop bleeding after a tooth extraction. It is also recommended as a douche for leucorrhoea.

LAVENDER

LAVENDER   *Lavandula angustifolia* Mill.
                                                    LABIATAE

Lavender is controlled by the planet Mercury, under whose dominion is the nervous system. This plant is the "Nardus" of the Greeks, named for the Syrian city Naarda, on the Euphrates River. It is often referred to in old books as "Nard," and St. Mark called it "spikenard." Pliny said that it sold for as much as one hundred Roman "dinari" a pound, which in our money would be roughly ten dollars.

Lavender's volatile oil contains over one hundred components.

It is aromatic, carminative, and, not surprisingly as it is under Mercury, a nervine.

Herbalists today use lavender in the treatment of headache, sunstroke, weakness and swelling of the limbs, and to control vomiting and hysteria. The usual dose is a cupful of the infusion (standard brew) made from the flowering spikes, fresh or dried.

Lavender bags are placed among linens and clothing as both perfume and moth repellent. Flies and mosquitoes dislike the fragrance, which we find attractive; so a vase of cut flowers which includes sprigs of lavender can be practical as well as beautiful.

Culpepper said the flowers steeped in wine "help those to make water that are stopped, or troubled with wind or colic, if the place be

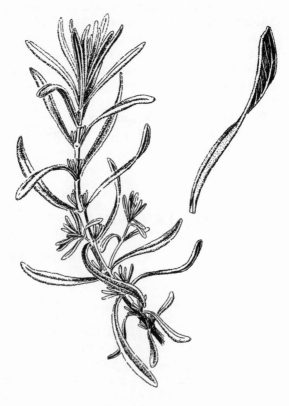

Lavender

bathed therewith," and "to gargle the mouth with a decoction thereof, is good against the toothache."

I steep lavender spikes in cider vinegar, add a little orange-flower water, and use it as a skin tonic. A decoction of cucumber juice and lavender makes another good skin lotion. If you prefer a cream, mix either one with melted cold cream; then allow to cool.

A fomentation of lavender as external application relieves local pains and stiffness of the joints.

During both World Wars, lavender was used to cleanse wounds, and the oil is presently being tried as a surgical dressing.

Veterinarians in England use lavender oil to get rid of lice and other animal parasites. I put lavender in my dog's bath water as a preventive after he has been running in the woods.

Oil of lavender is sometimes effective in bringing back circulation to feet that have lost feeling. Whether or not it is effective depends on the cause. It is harmless, so try it; if it doesn't work, consult your doctor for a diagnosis.

In gardens, lavender grows well in sandy or limestone soils. It is easily started from root division or from seed. In northern Vermont the plants grow to eighteen inches high, branching out widely. They prefer a sunny well-drained place shielded from the prevailing west wind. Sessile leaves are opposite, thin, blunt, grayish, slightly revolute or rolled back from the margin. The terminal flower spikes hold whorls of six to ten bluish-purple, lipped blossoms. The calyx contains the aromatic oil in its glands.

Plants are apt to get woody after three or more years, so it is a good plan to start new ones every second year.

LEMON BALM

LEMON BALM
("MELISSA")

Melissa officinalis L.

LABIATAE

This fragrant perennial grows happily in most parts of the world: Europe, Asia, North and South America, and landfalls in between. Its botanic name, *Melissa,* came from the Greek word for bee, a reminder of

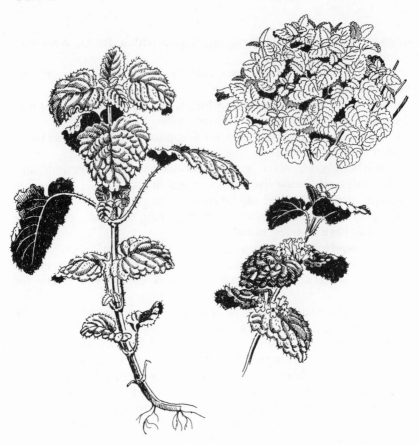

Lemon Balm

the fondness bees have for the honey produced by the plant. Pliny, addressing himself to bee-keepers said, "When they are strayed away, they do find their way home by it."

Its popular name, balm, was an abbreviation of balsam, which refers to a plant or tree yielding a balsam, or "any agency that heals, soothes or restores."[1]

Melissa grows up to two feet high; its opposite leaves are heart-shaped, the edges finely toothed. Bruise a leaf and you will notice a sweet,

---

[1] *Random House Dictionary of the English Language,* The Unabridged Edition. New York: Random House, 1966.

lemony fragrance. It is not fussy about soil and will grow well in any garden. It can be started from seeds, cuttings, or root divisions. The serrated leaves are attractive; it is a neat, bushy plant which holds its shape, attracts bees, and is useful as a pleasant addition to our cuisine as well as for a medicine. It is carminative, diaphoretic, febrifuge, vulnerary, and disinfectant.

Carmelite water, which consisted of lemon balm as the principal ingredient as well as lemon peel, nutmeg, and angelica root, once had a reputation for curing nervous headache and neuralgia. Charles V, also known as Charles I of Spain, drank carmelite water every day during the fifty-eight years of his life. Son of Philip the Fair of Flanders and Joanna the Mad of Spain, Charles may have been protected from hereditary madness by the balm. In any case, it probably added to its reputation for so doing because John Evelyn wrote, "Balm is sovereign for the brain, strengthening the memory and powerfully chasing away melancholy."

Both Pliny and Dioscorides believed that "Balm, being applied, doth close up wounds without any peril of inflammation." Today science has "discovered" that the balsamic oils of many aromatic plants make effective surgical dressings because of their ability to give off ozone and thus prevent putrefaction.

Paracelsus called *Melissa* the "elixir of life."

Balm is also useful as a tea to cool the temperature of patients suffering from influenza or other chills-and-fever type infections. Use a standard brew and administer one-half cupful at a time, warm, every few hours.

Another use I have found for *Melissa* is to put a bruised leaf inside a bandage or band-aid to heal stubborn cuts.

Less medicinally, but more socially, lemon balm is a delicious addition to a claret cup. Combine a handful of balm, a few borage leaves, a thin-sliced lemon and orange, a shot glass of cognac, a half cup of honey, a bottle of claret and a pint of seltzer water or any good brand of carbonated water. Let stand with enough ice to cool, strain, and decorate with the blue, star-shaped blossoms of borage.

A fine home-made liqueur can be made by taking two handfuls of crushed *Melissa* leaves, putting them in a glass jar or crock, pouring over them a fifth of vodka, three-quarters cup of honey, and a grated lemon peel. Shake well and let stand for a week. Strain, bottle, and test your character by waiting three weeks before using.

This is a basic recipe which I use to make other herbal liqueurs as well as the popular Mexican cordial, Kahlua. For the latter, use two vanilla beans, one cup of strong black coffee, one cup of honey, and a fifth of vodka. Let the mixture stand, unstrained, for one month.

MALLOW

HIGH MALLOW	*Malva sylvestris* L.
COMMON MALLOW	*M. neglecta* Wallr.
("CHEESES," "LOW MALLOW")	
MARSH MALLOW	*Althaea officinalis* L.
HOLLYHOCK	*Alcea rosea* L.
	MALVACEAE

The *Malvaceae* comprise nearly one thousand species, which are distributed from the tropics to the arctic, the number decreasing as they go north. All species are emollient and demulcent in varying degrees, and some are expectorant and diuretic. They contain starch, mucilage, pectin, oil, sugar, asparagine, phosphate of lime, glutinous matter, and cellulose. The family name *Malvaceae* comes from the Greek word "malake," or soft, as the plant heals and soothes.

The mallows are useful in treating sore throats and laryngitis, and as a soothing demulcent for the lining of the stomach. Their emollient qualities make them helpful for skin irritations and insect stings.

The fresh, young leaves and the whole seed pod are edible. The latter is often referred to in country places as "cheese." In countries where crop failures often bring famine, the mallows are an important subsistence food. The roots may be boiled, or steamed, then panfried with butter or oil and onions.

An infusion of *Malva* species was used in combination with chokecherry gum by the Arikara Indians of Michigan to control postpartum hemorrhage.

In France, a confectioners' paste, *pâté de guimauve*, is made from the roots of the marsh mallow. But the marshmallows sold in the United States are made from flour, gum, and egg albumin and contain no mallow.

The garden hollyhock is usually considered a decorative companion to old, dry stone walls and white picket fences, but the flowers, the part used, are very helpful in treating chest and lung congestion. *Alcea rosea* is diuretic as well as emollient and demulcent.

Mallows have been used medicinally from early times by the Arabs, the Greeks, and the Romans, and are used today as food and medicine by herbalists everywhere.

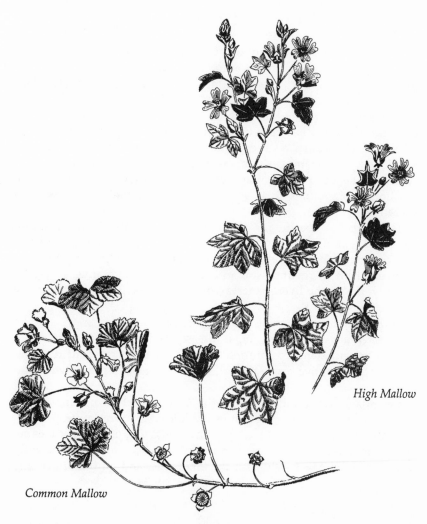

High Mallow

Common Mallow

Mallows

MEADOWSWEET

MEADOWSWEET *Filipendula ulmaria* (L.)
Maxim.[1]

ROSACEAE

The phrase "a rose by any other name would smell as sweet" certainly applies to meadowsweet. It has been called by many names referring to its species, but no one (so far) has challenged its generic place in the rose family.

Its virtues have been known since the time of Dioscorides. Its pharmaceutical largesse has been buttressed by a series of scientific discoveries, and laboratory tests continue to unravel its chemical secrets. Meadowsweet contains calcium, magnesium, sodium, and sulphur, salicylic acid, heliotropin, vanillin aldehyde, and a few, so far unnamed, additional compounds. It is astringent, diuretic, tonic, nutritive, and alterative.

This herb is a specific for diarrhea in children; its astringent action combined with nutritives makes it safe, mild, and effective. Its salicylic acid content makes it useful in treating influenza, respiratory tract infections, arthritis, rheumatism, and fevers. As an alterative, meadowsweet works on the liver, pancreas, and intestines. It causes food to be digested easily.

Flowers and leaves made into an infusion, standard brew, may be taken internally for all the above diseases and as a blood purifier. A double-strength standard infusion, taken cold, is an excellent tonic for pre- or post-operative cases, general convalescence, or a run-down condition.

Gerard, in 1597, called this herb "Mede-sweet or queene of the medowes." I like his description of it, valid and appreciative.

"This herb hath leaves like Agrimony, consisting of divers leaves set upon a middle rib like those of an ash tree, each small leaf slightly snipt about the edges, white on the inner side, and on the upper side

---

[1] Formerly *Spiraea ulmaria* L. *Spiraea latifolia,* an American species, is a legitimate entity completely distinct from *Filipendula ulmaria* (L.) Maxim. (*Spiraea ulmaria* L.)

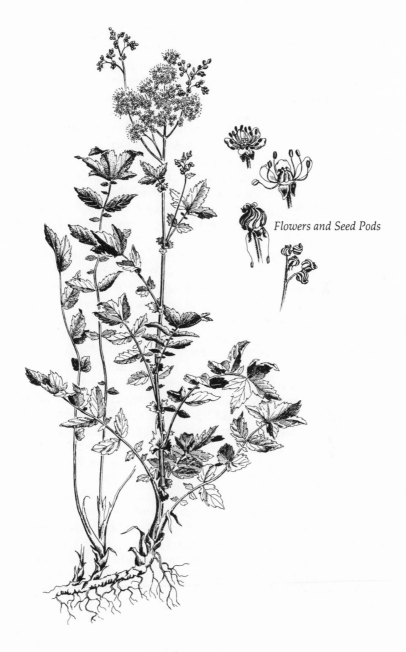

Flowers and Seed Pods

Meadowsweet

crumpled or wrinkled like unto those of the Elm tree; wherof it took the name Ulmaria, . . . The stalke is three or four foot high, rough, and very fragile or easie to be broken, of a reddish purple colour: on the top whereof are very many little floures clustering and growing together, of a white colour, . . . and of a pleasant sweet smell, as are the leaves likewise.

"It groweth in the brinkes of waterie ditches and rivers sides, and also in medowes. . . . It is called Regina prati: in English Meads-sweet, Medow Sweet, and Queen of the Medowes."

Some fifty years later Culpepper gave a similar, albeit more technical, description and gave its name as *Spiraea ulmaria*. This was the official name of the plant in 1827, when a French chemist, searching for the active pharmaceutical ingredient of the willow, isolated salicin from meadowsweet.

In America, as late as 1944, *The New Garden Encyclopedia* defined meadowsweet as the "common name for three species of *Spiraea* namely, *S. alba, S. latifolia,* and *S. saliciflera* or *salicifolia. S. alba* and *S. latifolia* are now said to be the same plant. The name is also sometimes applied to *Filipendula,* a genus of hardy perennials." Under *Filipendula* the *Encyclopedia* has this to say, "A genus of hardy perennial herbs of the Rose family resembling certain Spiraeas." It lists *F. ulmaria* as the Queen of the Meadow, calling it an escape in the eastern states.

Two other varieties of spiraea are called meadowsweet in common usage. One is hardhack, *Spiraea tomentosa,* which is native to America. It was used by various Indian tribes, and a nineteenth-century doctor, Francis Porcher, called it a valuable tonic and astringent useful in diarrhea. Its leaves were used by the Mohegans to cure dysentery; the Ojibwa Indians made a tea of leaves and flowers to cure morning sickness and to facilitate parturition.

Spiraea salicifolia, called the willow-leaved meadowsweet, was used medicinally by the Potawatomi Indians and by white frontier doctors.

Filipendula ulmaria, as well as other herbs called meadowsweet, have proven valuable during food shortages because of their nutritional content, which includes minerals vital for good health—calcium, magnesium, and sodium. They are also valuable to rebuild tissue and are used to treat anemia.

MILK THISTLE

MILK THISTLE   *Silybum marianum* (L.) Gaertn.
COMPOSITAE

I fell in love with milk thistle years before I planted it in my garden. It grew along the ditches on the winding roads from Camino de las

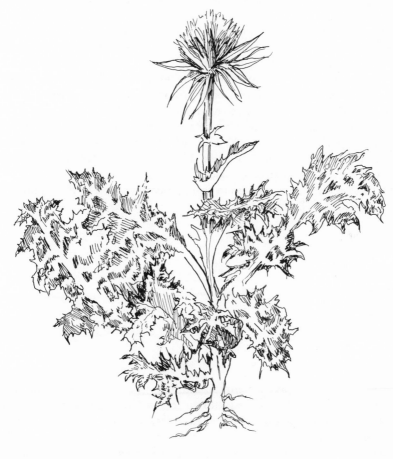

Milk Thistle

159

Huertas to the olive orchards on the hills beyond. The deeply cut leaves of generic green were bright with carefree-spilled white swirls, so rhythmic in their clasparound strong stems that the terminal purple blossoms were almost anticlimactic. A strong plant with a good self-image, it sent out a clear message. "I am important; get to know me." I tried. In Villa Nueva, however, no one knew its name. "Cardo," just "thistle." But in Madrid I rushed to the Library of the Botanical Garden and found its name: *Silybum marianum*. Two years later I talked to herbalists in Spain and in France. I made an impressive list. This self-assured "cardo" had always been used to cure mushroom poisoning and liver malfunctions, and to prevent harm from pollutants, agricultural or industrial wastes, and "bad water."

Now milk thistle has its place in my garden. Like rosemary and lady's mantle, it brings a mythic background. Mary, it is said, sat among green thistles to nurse the infant Jesus and spilled milk on the leaves.

Whole seeds or a tincture made from them are now used in the United States as well as in Europe, for both protection and regeneration of the liver. Powdered seeds are also available in capsules.

Fresh seeds from the plant can be gathered for use as a healthy food. Toasted in a skillet, they can be crushed and sprinkled on other foods.

Silymarin, a constituent of milk thistle, is now listed in *The Merck Index* as a liver protector. No toxicity has been reported from the use of milk thistle, but our advice, as in trying any new food or drug plant, is to start with small amounts.

MULLEIN

MULLEIN   *Verbascum thapsus* L.
                                    SCROPHULARIACEAE

The tall, velvet-leaved biennial, mullein, is under the protection of the planet Saturn. It was well known to the Greeks, who made lamp wicks of its dried leaves, and to the Romans, who dipped its dried stalk in tallow for funeral torches.

Mullein belongs to a large family comprising some two hundred genera, within which there are nearly fifteen times that many species.

Two of the best known are garden penstemon and foxglove. John Burroughs, assiduous nineteenth-century plant watcher, gives his observation of mullein, "The first year it sits low upon the ground in its coarse flannel leaves, and makes ready; (if the plow comes along its career is ended). The second season it starts upward its tall stalk, which in late summer is thickly set with small yellow flowers, and in fall is charged with myriads of fine black seeds."

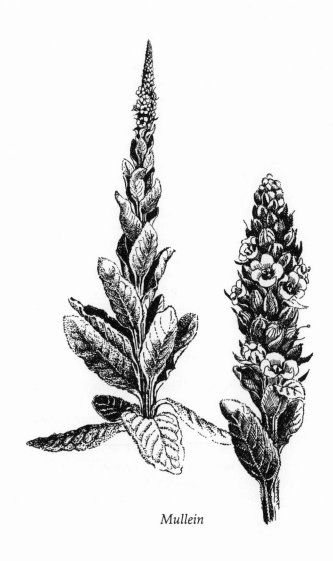

Mullein

The leaves of mullein are mucilaginous, taste bitter, and contain gum, resin, a yellow coloring principle, a somewhat fatty chlorophyll, a glucoside, some acrid fatty matter, free acid and phosphoric acid, noncrystallizing sugar, mineral salts with potassia and lime bases, and a small amount of yellowish volatile oil.

The plant is demulcent, emollient, and astringent, which makes it a valuable herbal remedy for pectoral complaints and any bleeding from lungs or bowels. The entire plant is sedative and anodyne, a non-narcotic pain killer.

Dry or fresh leaves, boiled for ten minutes in one pint of milk and strained, can be taken warm, with or without honey, as a nutritive medicine. This is also helpful for coughs or hemorrhoids.

For diarrhea in adults or children, add a fresh leaf or one teaspoon of ground dried leaf to one pint of warm milk to which honey and nutmeg or ginger have been added. The dose is one-quarter cup every fifteen minutes for two doses, then every half hour until the mixture is finished.

The lower leaves may be used externally, mashed in cider vinegar, for relief of swollen glands, tonsils, and asthma. The dried leaves smoked in a pipe are also good for asthma, a method used by the Potawatomi.

I put dried leaves in an enamel pot, cover them with water and bring to a boil, then breathe in the fumes with a towel over my head to hold the steam in, for nasal and bronchial congestion.

The Menominee Indians smoked the root for pulmonary diseases. Other tribes made a smoke smudge which they inhaled for curing catarrh and to revive an unconscious patient.

The fresh leaves, macerated in olive oil, put in a corked bottle, and kept in a warm place for several days, make a good local application to be used for piles, frostbite, and for bruises or any mucous membrane inflammation. The fresh flowers, soaked in olive oil for three weeks, are effective as a bactericide.

Nicholas Culpepper says that, "The juice of the leaves and flowers laid on rough warts, as also the powder of the dried roots rubbed on, takes them away." Mullein leaves and flowers were officially in the *National Formulary* from 1916 until 1936.

I have several mullein plants in my garden where their stately velvet towers form a handsome background for smaller herbs, and a convenient source of medicine. This takes them out of the "weed" category, if we accept the definition of a weed as "A plant that grows where you don't want it!"

PLANTAIN

COMMON PLANTAIN   *Plantago major* L.
  ("BROAD-LEAVED PLANTAIN")
RIBWORT   *Plantago lanceolata* L.
  (NARROW-LEAVED PLANTAIN,
  "ENGLISH PLANTAIN")

PLANTAGINACEAE

Over two hundred species of plantain grow throughout the world.
The two most common plantains in the United States are *P. major* and

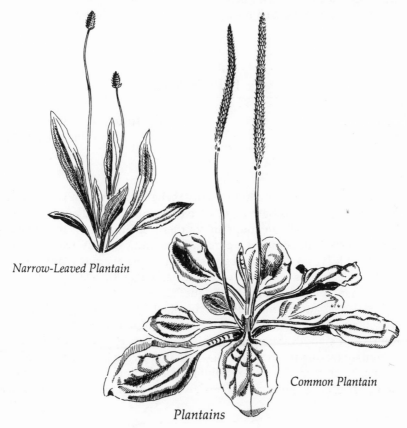

Narrow-Leaved Plantain

Common Plantain

Plantains

P. lanceolata, the broad-leaved and the narrow-leaved. The roots are long, straight, and difficult to dig out of lawns. A long slender spike bearing greenish or purplish flowers grows out of a rosette of leaves close to the ground. It is, of course, very perennial!

An important constituent of plantain is the glucoside aucubin. The herb is refrigerant, diuretic, vulnerary, deobstruent, and astringent. The macerated fresh leaves are put on bee stings, and used for skin irritations, malignant ulcers, and burns, and to stop bleeding in minor cuts.

Plantain was one of the nine sacred herbs of the ancient Saxon Lacnunga in which it is called "Weybroed." Its healing qualities are mentioned by Chaucer and Shakespeare.

A very effective salve can be made from southernwood, plantain, black currant and parsley leaves, and the buds and leaves of elder. Good for burns and raw surfaces.

An infusion, standard brew, is a mild cure for diarrhea.

PURSLANE

PURSLANE *Portulaca oleracea* L.
PORTULACEAE

Purslane, herb of the Moon, is an excellent food which is sold in the markets of Mexico as both a pot herb (like spinach) and a salad herb. It is used as salad and in soups in southern Spain and on the island of Crete, where it is raised as a garden plant and carefully watered, as its succulent leaves require more moisture than the average plant. Perhaps because it absorbs so much water, it "assuages thirst," as Culpepper said, when "placed under the tongue."

The leaves are round, fat, succulent; it lies on the ground, never stretching up to more than four to six inches. The reddish stems are round and smooth. Many vegetable gardeners consider it a weed, assiduously tearing it out when they find it growing between the rows. It should be cherished; cut carefully, it will continue to produce its delicious, refreshing leaves and stems all summer. As the roots grow near the surface, they will not interfere with other crops and will conserve moisture in the soil.

In ancient times purslane was considered a protection against magic. Since then, its value as a food providing the same diet additions as spinach, sorrel, and dandelion greens (choline and inositol) has been recognized.

The bruised leaves placed on the forehead will relieve a headache, particularly if caused by heat or lack of sleep. Eaten raw, it is good for the teeth and recommended for shortness of breath. Externally, the raw leaves are soothing to inflammation of the skin.

Take a few sprigs of purslane when going on a long hike. It will allay thirst if you chew it occasionally, and it is easier to carry than a thermos jug.

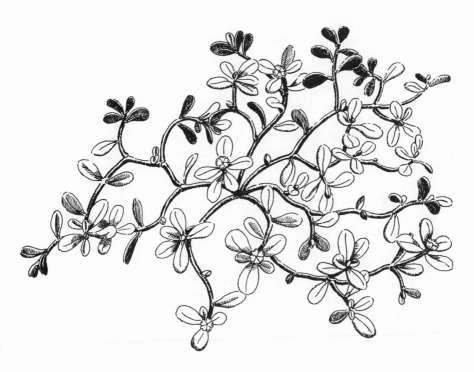

Purslane

165

ROSEMARY

ROSEMARY   *Rosmarinus officinalis* L.

LABIATAE

Rosemary, under the dominion of the Sun, is a warmth-loving plant which gives to our brain and body both stimulation and heat. Externally it is used as a skin lotion and a fragrant addition to bath water; as a hair rinse it stimulates follicle health and prevents baldness.

Rosemary contains tannic acid, resin, a bitter principle, and a volatile oil. It is antispasmodic, stimulant, stomachic, and astringent. It has in the past been used as an emmenagogue and chologogue, but we do *not* recommend the oil in these two uses for home treatment because an overdose could cause poisoning. Therefore, we will limit our discussion of rosemary's very important contributions to external treatment and culinary use.

The leaves, simmered in wine, are an excellent external application for rheumatic pains, sores, eczema, bruises, and wounds.

Infused as a standard brew, rosemary is an antiseptic mouthwash, pleasant to the taste.

In our northern garden, rosemary is a short, spreading, shrubby plant with opposite leathery, dark green leaves, shiny above and downy gray-white beneath with entire, pointed, linear, slightly rolled edges. Pale blue-to-lavender flowers grow in short, axillary racemes. In Vermont, rosemary does not bloom until July or August. In cold climates it is a tender perennial which must be potted and taken in for the winter. Once in the house, it does best in a cool location, and the soil should be allowed to dry out completely before it is watered. Then it should be soaked thoroughly so the roots will not come to the surface for moisture. Wash the leaves once a month with a bath of room-temperature water and castile soap suds. Do *not* use a detergent.

The dried leaves, smoked as tobacco, are helpful for coughs, bronchitis, and asthma.

Rosemary is a natural insecticide and protects other plants by its friendly presence. A standard brew may be used to bathe the skin when gardening during the mosquito, May-fly, or deer-fly season.

On the island of Crete, I learned to use fresh rosemary leaves and lemon juice to baste chickens turning on an outdoor rotisserie. The result is a culinary delight.

In many European and Central American cities, pharmacies in older sections still sell "Hungary Water," or "Queen of Hungary Water"—a toilet water used for faintness—as a skin bracer, body perfume, and application for headaches. It is also used in an atomizer as an air purifier. The flowering tips of rosemary are the therapeutic ingredients.

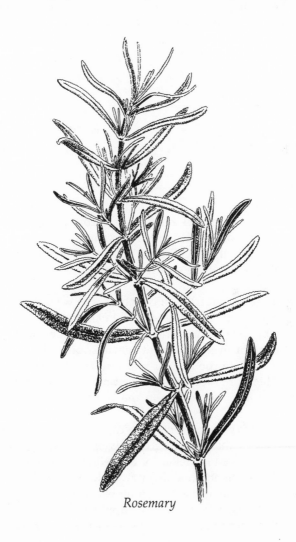

Rosemary

In southern Spain, rosemary is used as a disinfectant for wounds and, in powdered form, to heal babies' navels after the umbilical cord has been tied. Now that home deliveries in the United States are becoming popular again, I hope that young mothers and mid-wives will use this readily available and effective antiseptic.

In its native habitat along the rocky coasts of the Mediterranean, rosemary is not the tender little garden plant that we are familiar with. It grows to be a tall, spreading shrub, its roots happy with a thin layer of dry soil and its leaves refreshed with sea spray.

RUE

RUE   *Ruta graveolens* L.
("HERB OF GRACE")

RUTACEAE

Rue is a shrubby perennial, blue-green in color, forming a neat, perfectly rounded mass of leaves divided into tripinnate-rounded sections. Its lapis-lazuli tones, slightly silvered, make it a gem-like contrast to the other vegetable greens of the garden. Its greenish-yellow flowers grow in terminal panicles.

A native of the Mediterranean countries, rue was known to the ancient civilizations; Mithridates used it as an antidote for poisons. It was respected as a protection against witchcraft and believed to impart second-sight. No proof of second-sight remains, but Pliny reported that painters of his day ate rue regularly to restore overstrained eyes.

The name "herb of grace" reflects the time when a brush of rue was used to sprinkle the holy water in the ceremony "Asperges" before High Mass.

It has been used to ward off contagious disease for centuries. Along with garlic, it was one of the active ingredients in the "Vinegar of the Four Thieves," which allowed the felons of Marseilles to rob the bodies of the dead without becoming infected themselves during the plague of 1722.

In our own time, rue is used as an herbal remedy to allay the pains of sciatica. The bruised leaves may be applied directly to the affected part, but the skin should be oiled protectively first. Fresh leaves applied to the temples relieve headache, and compresses saturated with a strong decoction can be applied to the chest to control bronchitis.

Rue contains caprinic, plagonic, caprylic, and œnanthyeic acids and a yellow crystalline substance called rutin. Its action is stimulating, antispasmodic, emmenogogic, stomachic, and somewhat emetic. For this reason it should not be taken after eating.

Rue is useful in treating coughs, colic, and flatulence. Externally it is an active irritant or rubefacient, which accounts for its action in treating sciatica.

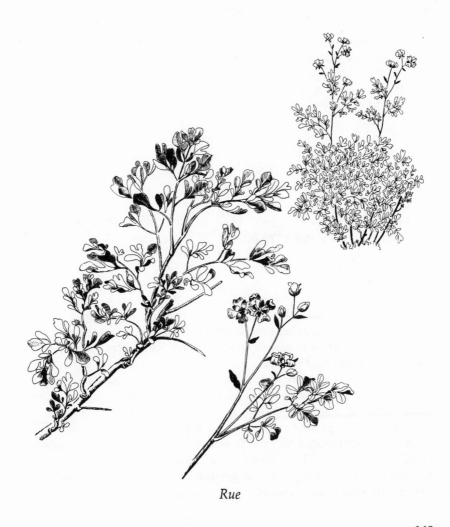

Rue

Like pennyroyal, rue is a good ingredient to put in water for mopping if you have pets. It will dispose of fleas and is harmless to animals.

An attractive sandwich can be made by rolling thin slices of bread spread with cream cheese and finely chopped young rue leaves.

We have been told that very occasionally rue may cause skin irritation by contact. I pass this warning on to you, but I have never seen a case of this sensitivity to rue in any of the hundreds of people who have been through my garden.

Rue grows readily from seed sown directly in the garden or started indoors. It can also be grown successfully from cuttings or root divisions. In the harsh winters of northern New England, it is surer to survive in relatively poor soil. All my soil is rich but well drained (my garden is on a hillside), but I throw a bit of sand and rubble around my rue plants in November. So far, my plants have lived through the winter; but as all gardeners know, there can always be that unprecedented first time.

SELF-HEAL

HEAL-ALL   *Prunella vulgaris* L.
("CARPENTER'S HERB")

LABIATAE

A hardy perennial, which sometimes grows to six or eight inches, self-heal is often procumbent and creeping. Its opposite leaves are round, slightly dentate, bract-like, with lavender-to-violet flowers growing from the axils in untapered spikes.

Prunella grows along roadsides, in lawns, meadows, wastelands, near stream banks, and near the edge of wooded areas. It is found all over North America, naturalized from Europe and its native Asia.

Linnaeus changed the original name, *Brunella*, to the softer sounding *Prunella*. Parkinson said that the Germans named it *Brunella* "because it cureth that disease which they call 'die bruen' (quinsey), common to soldiers in camp, but especially in garrison, which is an inflammation of the mouth, throat and tongue."

Prunella contains a volatile oil, a bitter principle, tannin, and sugar cellulose. It is astringent, styptic, and tonic.

In herbal medicine, prunella is used internally as a tonic prepared as a standard brew and taken, a wineglassful at a time, twice a day. Made into a syrup with honey, it is used for treatment of sore throat or ulcerated mouth.

The bruised, fresh leaves and flowers may be applied directly to a fresh wound. I have not found it so immediately effective as comfrey, yarrow, or bugle, but it is a good herb to know about because of its almost universal presence in city lawns as well as in country locales. One of its popular names, "carpenter's herb," indicates that its presence was known and gratefully used for many a mashed, bruised, or cut finger.

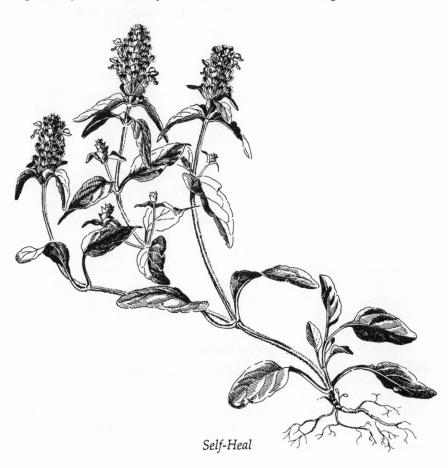

Self-Heal

SORREL

FRENCH SORREL	*Rumex scutatus* L.
SHEEP SORREL	*R. acetosella* L.
WOOD SORREL	*Oxalis* species
	POLYGONACEAE

The refreshing acidity or lemony taste of the sorrels is imparted by a salt—binoxalate of potash. The two varieties of the *Rumex* genus listed above are the most useful for menu and medicine, one wild, one cultivated. Both are diuretic, antiscorbutic, and refrigerant, excellent for cooling fevers, cleansing wounds, treating chronic skin diseases and urinary problems, and as blood purifiers.

French sorrel is a vigorous perennial plant for gardens. The large, pleasantly acid leaves may be chopped fine for salads or made into a delicious soup, which is equally good served hot or chilled. This is the way I make it:

Gather two large handfuls of sorrel. Wash, dry, and chop fine. Simmer in a large skillet with two tablespoons of butter until the sorrel has disintegrated. Add a tablespoon of flour, salt, and pepper to taste. Stir in and add one cup of soup stock (vegetable or chicken). Continue stirring until it thickens slightly. Remove from heat and add one cup milk or cream into which one egg yolk has been stirred. Return to the stove and stir while heating but do not allow to boil. Serve at once, hot, or refrigerate and serve chilled.

Quantities of this soup can be prepared in summer, frozen, and used in the winter. To do this, prepare as above until the soup stock has been added and brought to a boil. Then cool, put in a container, and freeze. When ready to use, defrost, add the milk or cream with egg yolk and serve.

When the stems of French sorrel grow tall, in mid-summer, cut the plant back, and new leaves will continue to grow until winter. Division of the roots in fall or early spring will insure a good supply each year.

Because of its food value, medicinal use, easy cultivation, and delicious taste, French sorrel is a plant that belongs in every garden.

Most of us who have walked through cool woods or along shaded paths know the delicate, acid wood sorrel, *Rumex acetosella*. The leaves are divided into three heart-shaped leaflets, light bright green above

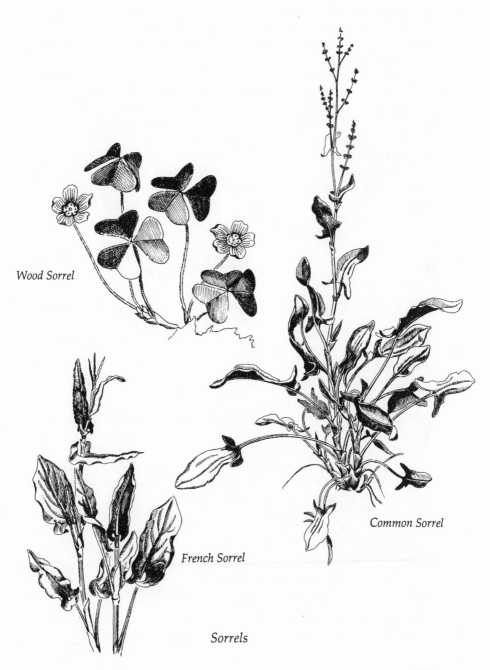

Wood Sorrel

French Sorrel

Common Sorrel

Sorrels

and violet tinged beneath with a crease or fold down the middle. The small, five-petalled white flowers are finely veined with purple. The leaves of this wild sorrel are smaller and thinner than the French sorrel, but can be used in the same way.

Sorrel leaves simmered in butter used to be a favorite green sauce for fish. I use it on steamed or broiled trout, perch, or red snapper.

Leaves of both French and wood sorrel can be used, fresh or dried, to make an infusion (standard brew), which may be taken, one-half cup three times a day, as a blood purifier. Externally, it can be applied as a wash or cold application to eczema or other skin irritations.

The sorrels, like the mints, the *alliums* (onions and garlic), and comfrey, should be included in everyday meals for maintenance of good health.

SWEET WOODRUFF

SWEET WOODRUFF   *Galium odoratum* (L.) Scop.
                        (*Asperula odorata* L.)
                                          RUBIACEAE

Sweet woodruff blooms in May in most climates, but in New England it is usually June before the small, white star-shaped flowers show above the narrow, light green leaves arranged around a stiff stem in whorls. About eight to twelve inches tall, it is a handsome border plant that retains its neat habit of growth and clear green color all summer.

Its medicinal qualities are many. Sweet woodruff is antispasmodic, antiseptic, anesthetic, astringent, diuretic, and tonic. Herbalists use it to treat nephritis, jaundice, and other diseases of the liver. An infusion is made of the whole herb, taken, a small cupful at a time, three times a day, before or after meals.

The action of sweet woodruff on the nervous system is that of a tranquilizer, one that is without side effects and is nontoxic. It helps cases of insomnia and is so gentle in its action that it can be used safely on the very old and the very young. It is also helpful in the treatment of colitis.

A household use of sweet woodruff is to perfume linen closets; the dried herb has the sweet scent of new-mown hay. In Scandinavian countries and in Germany it is an ingredient of fresh sausage, and in Alsace–Lorraine and Germany it is put in "May wine." The entire herb, leaves and flowers, is soaked in a sweet white wine for two weeks. The wine becomes slightly sparkling with an agreeable flavor and aroma, and is a good tonic. The bottle should be capped like champagne to prevent the cork from popping off.

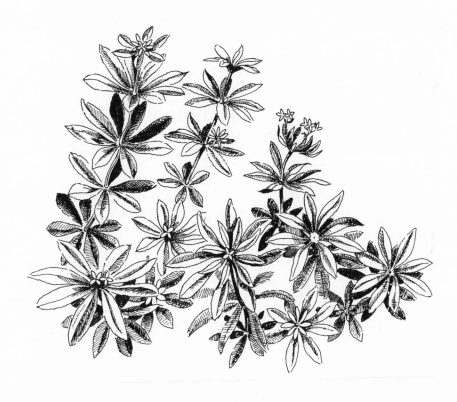

Sweet Woodruff

175

TANSY

TANSY   *Tanacetum vulgare* L.
                                             COMPOSITAE

Tansy, a hardy perennial ruled by Venus, grows to three feet high. The alternate leaves are cut in fern-like pattern, some six inches long and three to four inches wide. Round, flat, dull-gold flowers top the stems in late summer. The plant is easily recognized by its acrid but pleasant fragrance. It is found in abundance in waste places, in dry, poor soil. A nice garden variety is *crispum* which has leaves cut into finer, curled segments. This handsome plant does not bloom in my garden, so I also grow some of the wild plants. Both types will grow well in any garden soil, are easily increased by root division, in fact will spread naturally. Both wild and cultivated varieties have the same constituents: tanaceton, tannic acid, and a volatile oil (containing the toxin thujone). Tansy is anthelmintic, tonic, stimulant, and emmenagogic.

A popular remedy for worms in children, tansy was given as a tea (standard brew) night and morning on an empty stomach. In small doses it is stomachic, antiflatulent, and cordial. Tansy is a strong herb and should not be taken in large amounts. It should never be taken by pregnant women as it is abortifacient. In colonial times it was believed to cure sterility in women. It had another virtue, welcome before the age of refrigeration. It kept meat from spoiling. Culpepper said that, "if boiled in water and drank" it would ease griping pains and be good for sciatica and aching joints. It is also recommended for toothache and sore gums.

In England a traditional Easter dish was "a Tansy." The recipe is:

7 eggs, yolks and whites beaten separately
1 pint cream
1/4 to 1/2 cup spinach juice
a leaf of tansy mashed in a mortar
2 cups cracker crumbs (graham or soda crackers)
3/4 cup honey
a wineglassful of dry white wine
freshly grated nutmeg

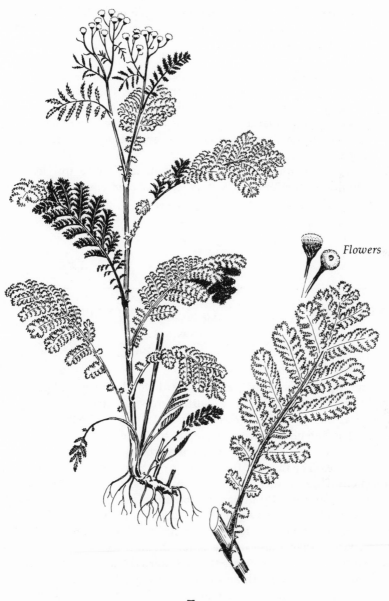

Flowers

Tansy

Combine all the ingredients, cook until thickened, cool slightly, and pour into a pie tin, lined with your favorite pie crust. Bake at 400° for fifteen minutes then reduce heat to 325° and cook until the custard is firm and a golden color.

Tansy was popular as a strewing herb because of its clean, acrid fragrance and because it kept flies and ants away. These qualities make it popular today, and it is frequently planted outside the kitchen door to discourage insects. Planted at intervals around the vegetable garden, along with wormwood, garlic, marigolds, and pennyroyal, it will discourage predatory insects.

Tansy has one other virtue which, in all fairness to this feathery plant, should be mentioned. A leaf, placed between your socks and the sole of your shoes, will prevent fatigue.

THYME

GARDEN THYME   *Thymus vulgaris* L.
                                        LABIATAE

Garden thyme has many branched, hard woody stems and grows to a height of about ten inches. The short, narrow, pointed leaves are only one-quarter inch long, dull green, growing in pairs on extremely short petioles. The lavender flowers terminate the branches in whorls.

Mother-of-thyme, *Thymus serpyllum*, is a prostrate, crawling plant with rounder leaves. The flowers, red-violet, grow between the paired leaves on the stem. Three attractive varieties for the garden are golden thyme, silver thyme, and woolly thyme, the botanical names for which are *T. vulgaris* aureus, *T. vulgaris* argenteus, and *T. lanicaulis*. The last has very woolly trailing branches which bloom early in the summer with pink flowers, larger than those of the other thymes. All varieties may be raised from seed, but the plants that are started from root division are usually hardier in the north and have a stronger fragrance.

The fragrance of thyme, like many of the *Labiatae*, attracts bees and gives a delightful flavor to their honey. Theophrastus boasted of the

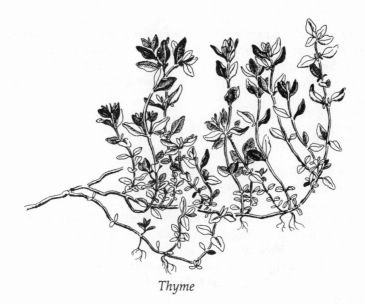

Thyme

superiority of honey in Attica, which owed its special quality to the wild thyme growing on Mount Hymettus. Virgil wrote of honey gathered from bees that fed on thyme, marjoram, and mother-of-thyme, "Fervet opus, redolenque Thymo fragrantia mella."

Thyme is antiseptic, antispasmodic, tonic, and carminative. It is used in treatment of whooping cough, colds, shortness of breath, and to clear the system of impurities. It is also good for fungus infections and sore throat. Gerard recommended it to "cure sciatica and pains in the head."

It is a safe and pleasant digestive taken in the form of an infusion (standard brew). Try these teas to keep your body in a state of health.

Equal parts of:
    Thyme, lavender, comfrey
    Thyme, mullein, red clover
    Thyme, rosemary, sage
    Thyme, comfrey, anise

Two parts thyme to:
    One part hyssop, and one part lovage

All species of thyme yield fragrant oils with thymol and carvacrol.

As a healthy culinary herb, thyme enhances the flavor of soups, stuffings, and home-made mayonnaise. It makes a fragrant herb butter to use on beets, carrots, or parsnips and is one of the herbs used with mace, allspice, parsley, and onions in Swedish meat balls.

Swedish Meat Balls
è.

Soak one-half cup of bread crumbs in two tablespoons of heavy cream. Add one-half pound ground pork, one-half pound of ground beef, 2 tablespoons minced onions, and rubbed spices to taste. Mix well, with salt and pepper to taste. Squirt into this mixture, a little at a time, approximately three-quarters cup of ginger ale or club soda. Add one beaten egg. Mix well again and shape into very small balls, not more than one inch in diameter. Fry lightly in butter and serve with whole cranberry or lingonberry sauce. Any leftover meat balls are delicious served cold as an hors d'oeuvre.

An herbal pipe tobacco can be made with equal parts of dried leaves of thyme, comfrey, mullein, and lovage. The well-blended herbs should be put in a tin with a slice of apple, tightly sealed and allowed to mellow for a month.

In the garden, thyme is a repellent for cabbage worms. Virgil, in his poetic advice to farmers, the *Georgics*, recommends thyme as a fumigant. Pliny said that when burned it discouraged "all venomous creatures."

WORMWOOD

WORMWOOD	*Artemisia absinthium* L.
ROMAN WORMWOOD	*A. pontica* L.
SOUTHERNWOOD	*A. abrotanum* L.
MUGWORT	*A. vulgaris* L.

COMPOSITAE

The *Artemisias* are under the dominance of the planet Mars, which gives to all living matter an energy of its own. They are bitter herbs.

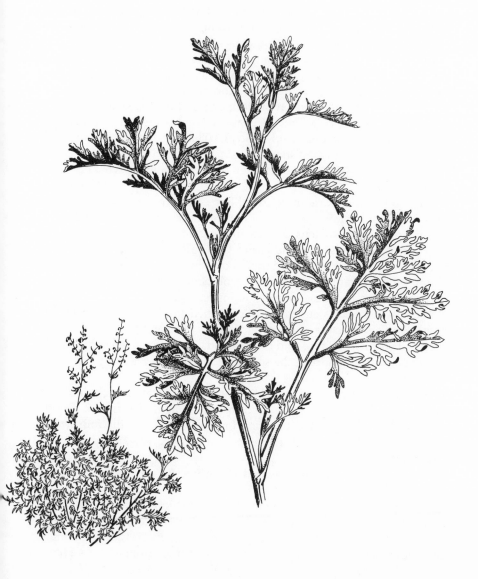

Wormwood

Wormwood is mentioned in the Bible, along with rue, and was used by the Jews as one of the bitter herbs eaten during the Passover.

Artemisia absinthium contains a volatile oil including thujone, thujyl alcohol, cadinene, phellandrene, and pinene, and the leaves contain the glucoside absinthin, absinthic acid, tannin, resin, starch, nitrate of potash, and other salts. It is aromatic, tonic, stomachic, febrifuge, anthelmintic, and antiseptic. It was listed in the *National Formulary* until 1926.

In ancient times, wormwood was used as an antiseptic to counteract the poisons of hemlock and some of the more deadly *Amanitas*.[1]

Tea made from an infusion of fresh or dried leaves, sweetened with honey, is a good spring tonic. It is also recommended after eating too much heavy food, as one is apt to do at a Thanksgiving dinner or other holiday meal. Wormwood should be steeped only five minutes because of the bitter taste instead of the fifteen to twenty minutes which is usual for herb teas.

All the artemisias are insect repellent; southernwood is particularly effective against moths. A swag of the fresh branches hung in a clothes closet will protect woolens. For use in my garden, I make an insecticide of wormwood, tansy, rue, and garlic. Chop all ingredients and steep in boiling water thirty minutes. Strain, cool, and apply in a spray gun to young cabbage, cauliflower, and broccoli plants. The spray will keep off all pests and is harmless to birds, animals, and humans.

Wormwood leaves cut fine and sprinkled in a circle around young plants is also effective. Cutworms can be held at bay by a circle of chopped wormwood tops and coarse sand. The bitter aroma of the herb and the abrasive texture of the sand will discourage the most rapacious worm.

Another use for wormwood has always been as an anthelmintic. To get rid of pin worms or thread worms, take one-half teaspoon wormwood in honey, night and morning for three days. On the fourth day drink an infusion of equal parts peppermint and yarrow, a cup morning and night.

Combined with rue, wormwood is a powerful antirheumatic treatment.

In America, the use of mugwort (*Artemisia vulgaris*) dates back to the seventeenth century. Captain Lawrence Hammond of Charlestown, Massachusetts, in his *Physical Receipts* listed mugwort, sage, chamomile, and gentian boiled in honey and applied warm, as a remedy. As I have

---

[1] Any agaracaceous fungus of the *Amanita group,* most of which are poisonous.

mentioned before, I do not agree with "boiling" honey. Put the raw honey in the hot decoction. In the early 1800's the Potawatomi of Wisconsin were using a wild wormwood (*Artemisia fridgida*) as a fumigant to revive patients from a coma. The plant is a source of camphor.

All of the artemisias are decorative in the garden because of their much-cut silvery leaves. Silver king (*A. ludoviciana* var. albula) grows in tall single stems with pure silver leaves, which are attractive in a summer bouquet and dry well for winter decorations. The neat, round, low-

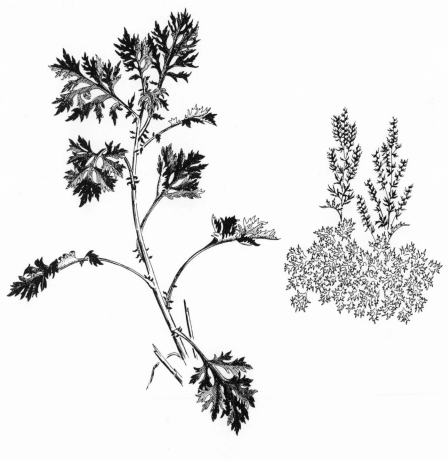

Mugwort

183

growing silver mound (*A. schmidtiana*) has feathery silver foliage and is a charming border plant.

Tarragon (*Artemisia dracunculus*) looks unlike other members of its family. Its narrow, dark green leaves are similar to hyssop or lavender. It does not set seed in the United States, but is easily propagated by root division in early spring or fall. In fact, clumps of the plant should be taken up and divided every third year, or the roots will strangle each other—the reason why the French name for tarragon is "estragon," Little Dragon.

I know of no medicinal use for this green member of the artemisia family, but its delightful flavor in vinegar, salads, and when cooked with chicken or veal, makes tarragon its own reward. It has some of the tonic and antiseptic qualities of its more powerful relatives, so it can properly be classed as a preventative herb.

The evening breezes . . .
Water lapping lightly on
the heron's leg-sticks

BUSON

September sunshine . . .
The hovering dragonfly's
Shimmering shadow

KARO

Autumn breezes shake
The scarlet flowers my poor child
Could not wait to pick

ISSA

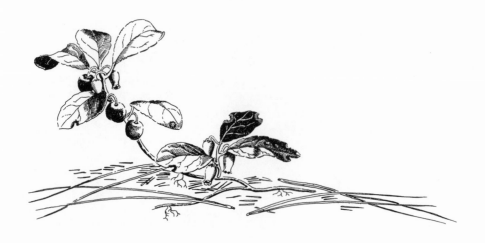

VIII

Autumn:
Battening Down

When the air is cool and crystal clear, and black and white cows, grazing a hill-pasture across the valley, are brought into sharp focus by a brilliant sun, the message our senses pick up is autumn. A day to walk along the river bank and throw a stout rope over butternut branches, to shake down the greenish-brown husks with sticky surfaces. We are not the only butternut seekers. Squirrels have their own way of knowing when it is time for gathering. Energy is high everywhere; flocks of birds, in traveling formation, make a "U" turn, swoop over harvested fields and head south.

We put our sack of butternuts in the woodshed. Taking a basket and a sharp-pointed spade, we go to dig roots of first-year burdock. In a brown paper bag we also gather seeds from last year's plants. The roots will be scrubbed, quartered, and dried to make blood-purifying teas. Seeds will be saved in jars against possible need in local applications for acne and psoriasis.

A few comfrey roots must be gathered too. And for elecampane, scouted in July, there is a hill where five or six plants were seen, tall and golden flowered.

After supper we make the first autumn fire in the living room stove; "Round Oak" throws out an encouraging warmth. We settle down in a comfortable chair and write on a lined yellow pad: bottle herbs, make salves, pot herbs for kitchen window, transplant herbs and vegetables into solar greenhouse, dig horseradish and jerusalem artichokes, pull up tomato stakes, roll up chicken wire from green peas, mark asparagus bed and rows of sorrel and parsnips with tall stakes that will show above the snow, put the garden to bed.

Now is the time to rub down and bottle those herbs, protected by paper bags, that have been hanging in the kitchen since August: agrimony, boneset, coltsfoot, comfrey, costmary, fireweed, goldenrod, lovage, mint, red clover, sage, vervain, and yarrow. They are all bone-dry now. Held over a large bowl, the leaves can be rubbed off the stems and the stems cut into small pieces. Clean jars should be lined up on the counter, a stack of labels waiting to be inscribed.

If you are drying and bottling your own herbs for the first time, use labels that are large enough for the following information: name of herb, common and botanical, date of bottling, and the condition the herb is used to remedy.

Coltsfoot-*Tussilago farfara*

23 September 1980

For coughs, sore throat, hoarseness
infusion, with honey
one cup, three or four times a day,
as needed

Making salves is a good occupation for a rainy day. The basic procedure is simple, traditional, but time-consuming.

Chop herbs. Put in an enamel or stainless steep pot. Barely cover herbs with spring, well, or bottled water. (Do not use highly-chemicalized city water.) Bring to a boil, let simmer thirty minutes. Strain. Add to liquid an equal amount of olive or safflower oil. Return to pot and simmer until all the water has evaporated. There will be no bubbles when the water is gone. Remove from fire and add enough beeswax to give the mixture a salve consistency. Put in a piece of wax about the size of a fifty-cent piece. Stir until dissolved. Pour a teaspoonful on a cool plate. If it thickens at once, the amount of wax is correct. If it does not thicken, quickly add more wax. Stir and bottle while hot. Label with date, ingredients, and use.

Two useful salves you might like to try are:

NUMBER 1

Two parts comfrey and/or plantain leaves
Two parts yarrow, leaves and flowers
One part St. John's-wort blossoms
One part pennyroyal and rosemary (whole herb)

This salve is useful for cuts, bruises, burns, and as a skin cream and lip salve.

NUMBER 2

Two parts cabbage leaves
Two parts mugwort and celandine (whole herb)
One part horsetail (*Equisetum arvense*), flowering thyme, and fireweed
    (*Epilobium angustifolium*)
One teaspoon ginger root or cayenne

This salve relieves muscular pains and discomfort due to bursitis or rheumatism.

Herbs for the kitchen window should be potted early in autumn. Clay pots are best as they are porous and will allow excess moisture to evaporate out. Place pebbles or broken bits of a clay pot in the bottom.

Fill with rich garden soil. Be sure roots are firmly tucked in. Water thoroughly with a dilute seaweed solution. Culinary herbs that grow well in the house, are fragrant, and add piquancy to winter cooking are: basil, chives, marjoram, rosemary, and thyme. Do not over-water; we all have a tendency to kill with kindness.

Rosemary will do well for me in the house until January. My opinion is that it needs a dormant season; so I water it heavily, cover it with plastic, and put the pot in a cool closet until April.

When selecting plants for the solar greenhouse, choose herbs and vegetables that are cold-resistant and have thick rather than thin leaves. Bibb lettuce, chinese cabbage, kale, leeks, parsley, winter savory, and salad burnet are good choices. The soil in the greenhouse should be very deep and rich. The bottom layer should be fresh manure, then layers of hay, wood ash, and top soil. When the planting is done, the soil should be moist. Water less frequently as the weather gets colder, and when the temperature goes down to ten degrees above freezing, stop watering. There should be enough condensation inside the glass to give the plants sufficient moisture. A top mulch of hay can be used but judge the condition of your own greenhouse; each one is different.

Horseradish roots may be dug any time before the ground freezes. Dig deeply because the roots are long. The root on one plant should be cut off one or two inches below the leaves. Return this small piece of root to the ground, press the soil around it firmly, and trim the leaves to about an inch above the ground. This will insure another crop of horseradish for next year.

Wash and scrub the roots and store them in the refrigerator in a plastic bag, well tied. Grate the roots as needed.

Jerusalem artichokes can also wait until late fall to be dug, after the small sunflower-like blossoms have come and gone. Unwashed, they keep well in a cool root cellar.

Putting the garden to bed is a chore that is pleasant; it keep you out of doors on cool sunny days, and the reward will be a painless spring with neat beds ready to plant and a minimum of pests who have wintered over, lurking in the soil.

Any unused herbs, leaves, and stems should be returned to the soil or added to the compost pile. Pull out by the roots all vegetables that have already been harvested: beans, broccoli, chard, cucumbers, cabbage. Pile them up away from the garden and chop well. Mix with dry leaves and a little hay and burn them if there is no local ordinance against this. In some towns permission must be obtained from the local fire warden. The ashes can be put in the compost pile, mixed with all surplus herbs.

Comfrey and sage leaves should be spaded into the soil. Both will discourage nematodes from spending the winter underground in the garden and improve your yield of tomatoes next year.

When all the trash is gone, mulch the whole garden with straw, grass clippings, or early hay that was cut before seeds formed.

Lemon, silver, and golden thymes, winter savory, lavender, and horehound do well with a light winter protection of spruce branches.

Asparagus beds should be fertilized with aged manure and compost each fall, then covered with mulch.

By Halloween our gardening will be finished, pumpkins and squash will be taken from the garden to a cool place, ready for use as baked vegetables, soups, bread, and pies. Halloween, or All Saints' Eve, was one of the two important Celtic festivals of the year, the other being May Day, or Beltane.

In the highlands of Scotland, it was the custom for children to gather ferns, and anything that would burn, and pile them into great heaps on a hill or rising ground near the house. At dusk these fires would be lighted, and the flames could be seen for miles around. Until the end of the eighteenth century, the ashes from these fires were gathered up and arranged in a large circle. Each member of the family or neighborhood placed a stone inside its circumference. Next morning the stones would be examined to see if any were displaced or missing; this would be interpreted as a sign of bad luck.

In the United States, herb gardeners who feel the urge to prepare for winter with a Halloween or autumnal bonfire may have a more direct connection with this ancient Celtic custom than is generally known. In the February Newsletter of the Vermont Academy of Arts and Sciences, anthropologist Lucien Hanks reviews Dr. Warren Cook's *Ancient Vermont*. One of the stone chambers discovered in Vermont, he says, "is aligned so that the winter solstice can be sighted at its doorway, suggesting a relationship to Stonehenge and other European remnants of Celtic times." Stone chambers found all over New England and other parts of the United States have been provisionally dated as before four hundred B.C.

Whatever the eventual opinion of the purpose of these stone chambers may be, it is safe to assume that our subconscious wish to burn summer's debris and to use fire as a purification rite before the seminal season of winter, goes very far back into the past of European and African cultures.

ALOE

ALOE *Aloe vera* L.
LILIACEAE

A native of Africa, *Aloe vera* has been naturalized in most of the tropical zones. In North America it grows only as a house plant. The long, succulent leaves are pointed and grow in rosette form. When broken, the leaves exude a thick, mucilaginous liquid which is very soothing and healing to burns and minor cuts. It relieves the pain immediately and heals if the application is repeated.

The plants require very little water. During the winter they can go for several months without being watered. They require small amounts during warm weather when they go into a period of growth. In the summer, small shoots which appear next to the mother plant can be removed and potted to form new plants. The large plants should be repotted into larger containers about every two or three years.

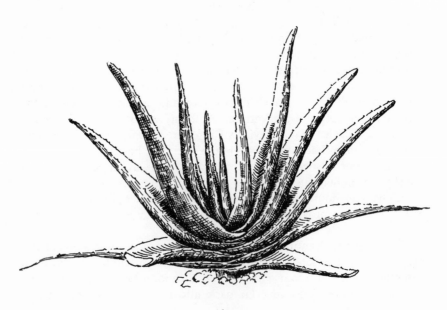

Aloe

The active ingredients of *Aloe vera* have not been identified as far as this author knows, but from personal observation and from consistent reports from persons who have used it as a treatment for burns, it is invariably effective.

The thick juice from a broken leaf may be rubbed on the skin as a beauty treatment. It nourishes the skin, and prevents and diminishes wrinkles. Wash the face with hot water and vinegar; then rub on the *Aloe vera* and allow it to remain on the skin all night.

BEARBERRY

BEARBERRY
("KINNIKINIC")

Arctostaphylos uva-ursi L.

ERICACEAE

Bearberry is a low, trailing, spreading, procumbent plant with small, spatulate, entire leaves with a leathery texture. They are a shiny dark green, finely veined. The berries are red and seem to be of interest only to bears and grouse. The flowers appear in drooping pink and white terminal racemes or panicles. In New England the blooming season is from June to July. It is usually found in dry, rocky, and sandy soil, but

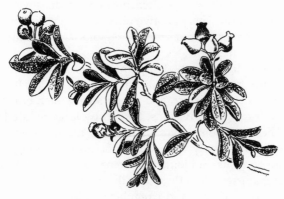

Bearberry

193

I have seen it growing contentedly along the edge of woods in moderately damp humus soil.

In the nineteenth century the plant was called *Arbutus uva-ursi* and is so classified in *Green's Universal Herbal*.

The leaves are the only part of the plant used medicinally.

Bearberry's main constituents are arbutin, methyl-arbutin, ursone, ericolin, gallic and tannic acids, and calcium oxalate. It is astringent, diuretic, antiseptic, soothing, tonic.

Uva ursi is used by both herbalists and the medical profession for treatment of such urinary problems as cystitis, urethritis, and nephritis. Youngken, in his *Text Book of Pharmacognosy*, lists it for these purposes.

Make an infusion of leaves, one ounce to one pint of boiling water and steep for twenty minutes. Marsh-mallow root can be combined in equal parts.

BONESET

BONESET   *Eupatorium perfoliatum* L.
("THOROUGHWORT")

COMPOSITAE

This hardy perennial was named for the Eupator of Pontus who, in 120 B.C. was Mithridates VI, whose extensive herb gardens were famous in the pre-Christian world. There are five hundred species of *Eupatorium*, many of which grow in warm or tropical regions. Over eighty species grow in the United States.

Boneset grows wild in low, damp meadows throughout North America as far south as Florida and also in the West Indies. It grows to four feet high with a strong, erect, and round stem which branches out at the top into four or more divisions, topped by large, white terminal flower heads. These are somewhat bristly with the hairs arranged in single rows. The plant is easy to recognize because the long, pointed, serrate leaves are opposite and joined at the base. The leaves of boneset are perfoliate, a characteristic reflected in the botanic name. The leaves have a prominent central vein and irregular veinlets.

Boneset is stimulant, febrifuge, diaphoretic, and laxative. It acts on the

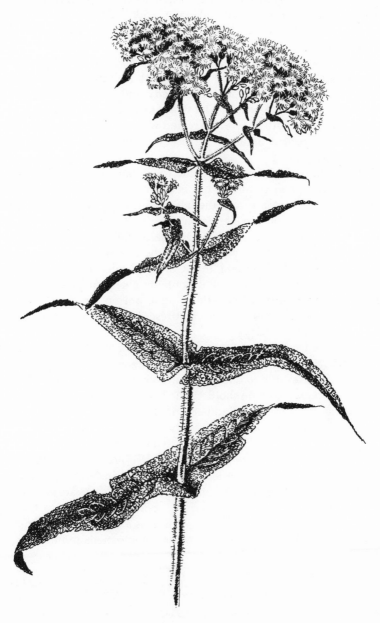

Boneset

stomach, liver, bowels, and uterus. The herb contains a bitter glucoside called eupatorin, resin, volatile oil, gallic acid, and a glucosidal tannin.

It is used by herbalists in cases of influenza, intermittent fever, and systemic colds.

Boneset and other species of *Eupatorium* were listed among the fifty-nine indigenous remedies used by the North American Indians. Indians of the northeast used it as a fever remedy and identified it by a name which signified "ague-weed." The white men learned to use it success-fully to cure intermittent fevers. Treated with boneset, this type of fever was non-recurrent, whereas a relapse was apt to occur when it was treated with quinine.

During the yellow fever epidemic in Philadelphia in 1793, boneset was used with good results. It has been mentioned by every writer on American *materia medica* from the late eighteenth century to the end of the nineteenth century. In *The People's Common Sense Medical Advisor in Plain English*, published in 1895, Dr. Pierce calls it tonic, diaphoretic, and aperient. He recommended taking one to four ounces of a boneset infusion. It was called, he said, the "Golden Medical Discovery," and he was "thoroughly satisfied that it contains chemical properties which neutralize and destroy miasmatic or ague poison which is in the sys-tem." To break up a child's fever, he prescribed four teaspoonsful three times a day for three days.[1]

During the Civil War, boneset was used as a febrifuge for treatment of Confederate troops. Both Indian and white men used it as a panacea for many illnesses due to dampness and exposure, and it was found in "every well-regulated household."[2] The Iroquois and the Mohegans used it to combat chills and fever, and among the Creeks it was used in steam houses for aches and pains of the hips.

For ninety-six years *E. perfoliatum* was listed in the *United States Pharmacopeia* and remained in the *National Formulary* until 1950.

The plants should be collected in late August in New England, when the flowers are first opened, as both leaves and blossoms are used medici-nally. If you cannot collect it yourself, order the dried herb from any reputable source listed in Appendix V, as it is a valuable addition to any home medicine shelf. I use the following combinations in infusions:

---

[1] R. V. Pierce, M.D., *The People's Common Sense Medical Advisor in Plain English*, 42nd Edition. Buffalo, N.Y.: World's Dispensary Printing Office and Bindery, 1895.

[2] Frances P. Porcher, *Resources of the Southern Fields and Forests—Being Also a Medical Botany of the Confederate States*. Charleston, S.C.: Evans and Cogswell, 1863.

One part boneset, one part comfrey, one part mint
One part boneset, one part chickweed, one part anise
One part boneset, one part catnip, one part sage
Sweeten with honey

Joe-Pye-weed, *Eupatorium purpureum,* is another valuable member of
the same family. It is astringent and diaphoretic. Its common name was
derived from an Indian of the northeast who was said to have cured
typhoid fever with it by inducing extreme sweating. It was also used by
the Indians as an antisyphilitic.

Both boneset and Joe-Pye-weed are common, handsome, wild plants,
with a long history of medical efficacy. I can personally recommend
boneset as a cure for dengue or break-bone fever, which I contracted
during a long stay in the West Indies.

BURDOCK

BURDOCK   *Arctium lappa* L.
                                                  COMPOSITAE

The botanic name *Arctium* is derived from the Greek word "arktos"
meaning bear, an obvious reference to the plants' rough-coated burrs.

Burdock, which enjoys the protection of Venus, is no stranger to even
the best-cared-for gardens, where it appears along paths and against
barns and out-buildings, not confining its habitat to ditches and country
roads. The tall, sturdy burdock has large, round, wavy leaves and purple
flowers that grow on circular heads.

In color the plant is dull grayed-green, the branched stem rising to
four or more feet from a biennial root. The lower leaves are amorphously
heart shaped, very large, sometimes up to sixteen inches long, the underside covered with down. As the leaves ascend the stem, they de-
crease in size and become ovate. Burdock blooms at summer's end, and
by September the tubular purple florets with their pale styles have
metamorphosed into the intransigent hooked burrs which adhere to
garden gloves, clothing, dogs, and horses' manes and tails with a nice
impartiality. The long, fleshy root is neutral brown outside and white

197

within. First-year plants have only basal leaves, the second year a pithy, reddish stem puts out wavy branches.

Aperient, chologogue, diaphoretic, diuretic, alterative, tonic, and demulcent . . . burdock, indeed, has something for everyone. A valuable quality which makes it a must for every home medicine cabinet is its efficacy as a blood purifier. It removes toxic substances from the system

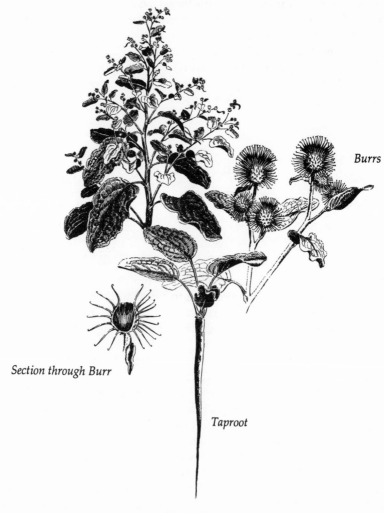

Burrs

Section through Burr

Taproot

Burdock

through action on the bile, kidneys, and sweat glands, relieving congestion of the lymph system. The root is the part most commonly used and should be collected in the spring or fall of the first year. A decoction of one teaspoon of the dried root, allowed to soak in an enamel pan for five hours (overnight would not be too long), then brought to a boil and strained, can be taken in the amount of one cupful a day. A supply for several days can be made and stored in the refrigerator. A standard decoction of the leaves is effective in the treatment of acne. An infusion of burdock leaves, one cupful a day, has long been used as a spring tonic.

Burdock, one of the most available plants, was well known to the American Indians. Vogel, in his book, *American Indian Medicine,* tells of four tribes who developed their own uses for it: the Otos, the Meskwaki, the Ojibwa, and the Potawatomi. They used it to treat pleurisy and combined it with other herbs to alleviate labor pains and to ease stomach cramps. The Potawatomi used the root very much as we do, as a blood purifier and tonic.

The white man learned about burdock from the Indians. It appeared in the *United States Pharmacopeia* intermittently from 1831 until 1916. It was not dropped from the *National Formulary* until 1947.

The root, in infusion or decoction, is recommended for skin diseases where purification of the system is indicated, such as in treatment of acne and eczema. This treatment is only effective, however, if the patient is willing to change his diet to one free of dairy products and to increase his intake of raw fruit and vegetables.

Burdock contains inulin, mucilage, sugar, a glucoside (lappin), a small amount of resin, fixed and volatile oils and some tannic acid.

CALENDULA

CALENDULA OR MARIGOLD   *Calendula officinalis* L.
COMPOSITAE

The familiar orange-flowered marigold received its botanical name because of its habit of blooming on the Calends, or first day of the month, according to the ancient Julian calendar. Its popular name "mari-

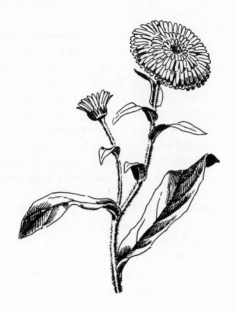

Calendula

gold" evolved from a corruption of the Anglo-Saxon "mersomeargealla," which actually referred to what we know as marsh marigold.

The green leaves of the *Calendula* or pot marigold are a bright, perfect green, prototype of what we envision the color green to be, neither dark, nor silvered, nor muted with any other tone, an equal mix of yellow and blue.

The medicinal properties of *Calendula officinalis* are antiseptic, stimulant, diaphoretic, febrifuge, mucilaginous, and vulnerary. The flowers are the part used. The plant is a source of organic iodine, which accounts for its antiseptic qualities. It prevents pus formation and promotes granulation of tissues to heal wounds and burns. As a vulnerary, a strong decoction, double the usual amount of herb to the usual amount of water, can be used warm or cool.

A lotion made from one cup of fresh blossoms simmered in two cups of milk is an excellent wash for the complexion. First, wash the face with natural (no preservatives) cider vinegar, let it dry on the skin, then dab on the calendula lotion.

A handful of blossoms steeped in a cup of olive or safflower oil, in a glass jar placed in a sunny window and turned occasionally, makes a therapeutic oil for sprains, congested veins, external ulcers, or skin problems. The oil may be left in the sun from one week to one month. The fresh flowers, bruised, may be applied directly to a cut or abrasion.

An infusion, standard brew, may be taken internally for treatment of low-grade fevers. It will also bring out the eruption in children's diseases, such as measles or chicken pox.

In medieval households the orange-colored blossoms were a standard ingredient of soups. The leaves, eaten in salads, were thought to be a cure for scrofula.[1]

Today we use the bright florets to give color to both soups and salads. To dry flowers, pull the petals apart and arrange them, without touching each other, on a large cookie sheet. If they overlap, the result will be blackening or loss of color. Dry in an oven that has been heated to two hundred degrees and then turned off. When the flowers are bone dry, store in a brown glass, ceramic, or stoneware jar. (The type of jar that cheddar cheese, or orange marmalade, comes in is excellent.) Besides adding color to winter stews and soups, the blossoms have some nutritional value. Dried calendula blossoms are also an economical substitute for saffron to color rice.

Pot marigold is an annual but will self-seed in good, loamy soil if weeded to give living space to the new, young plants. Under the influence of the Sun's purifying rays, the marigold embodies the quality of its patron and guardian.

The importance of marigold to the early colonists in New England may be judged by the fact that the seeds were among the first ordered by John Winthrop, Jr., as listed in the invoices of goods shipped in Captain Pierce's "Lyon." One-half ounce of marigold seeds cost, on the twenty-sixth of July, 1631, two pence, or "tuppence."[2]

Marsh marigold, which as we have mentioned gave its name to pot marigold by way of the Anglo-Saxon, is not a marigold, or a member of the *Calendula* family, but of the genus *Caltha* (*Caltha palustris*) of the buttercup family. It is a perennial with large, round, heart-shaped leaves, a hollow stem and flowers two inches across formed by yellow sepals rather than by petals. It grows in water or wet places and is a familiar sight in spring along ditches and in marshland. In Vermont, the early leaves have been used traditionally as an early spring green.

---

[1] A tuberculous disease characterized by swelling of the lymph glands, usually in the neck, and by inflammation of the joints.

[2] From the collection of the Winthrop papers, Volume III, Massachusetts Historical Society, Worcester, Massachusetts.

COHOSH

BLUE COHOSH   *Caullophylum thalictroides*
("PAPOOSE ROOT,"   Mich.
"SQUAW ROOT")

BERBERIDACEAE

Blue cohosh is found in rich, damp woods, often near streams. It grows two to three feet high with sheaving bracts at the base. Leaves are large, growing in threes on petioles. Each leaf is three-lobed near the apex. Flowers are six petaled, greenish to purple, and the berries are large and dry. The root, the part used medically, is thick, irregular, and knotty, with a brownish exterior, about four or five inches long with a white to yellowish interior.

Blue cohosh contains potassium, magnesium, gum, starch, salts, sodium, phosphoric acid, soluble resin, iron, silicon, a greenish-yellow coloring matter, and an ingredient corresponding in some ways to saponin.

It is diuretic, antispasmodic, tonic, stimulant (diffusive-relaxant), emmenagogic, diaphoretic, anthelmintic, parturient, antirheumatic.

It is used in the treatment of rheumatism, dropsy (excessive accumulation of serous fluid), and hysteria. It is an important herb during pregnancy and childbirth. Indian women drank the tea daily for several weeks before labor and for several hours before the actual birth, starting with the first labor pains. Taken during pregnancy, it strengthens the uterus. It brings on labor when the proper time has arrived and prevents it from being too prolonged or too rapid. It is also helpful for menstrual cramps.

DOSAGE

Infusion: One wineglassful three or four times a day, between meals
Decoction: One teaspoon to one tablespoon, three or four times a day

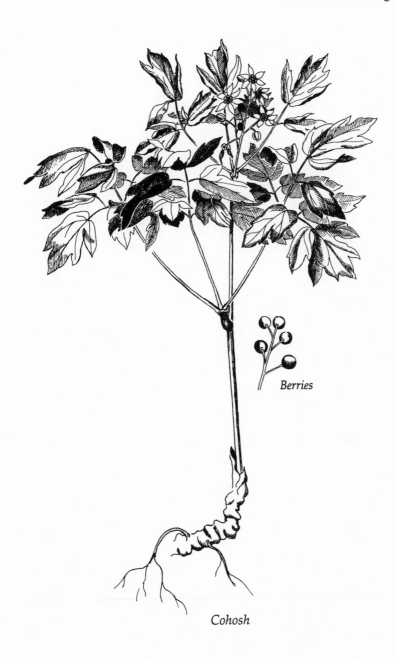

Berries

Cohosh

ELECAMPANE

ELECAMPANE   *Inula helenium* L.
                                                    COMPOSITAE

Elecampane, protected by the planet Mercury, is partial to damp pastures and somewhat shaded places. So adaptable is this four-to-five-feet-tall plant that it has made itself at home throughout Europe, temperate Asia, in southern Siberia, and parts of India, and is naturalized all over North America, where it is frequently seen growing along roadsides and in ditches and abandoned fields. The stout, erect stem branches out near the top, where it bears terminal heads of large, bright yellow flowers, four inches in diameter, which grow out of a base or involucre of wide velvety leaves (bracts). The leaves of the basal rosette are large, ovate, pointed, fifteen to eighteen inches long and up to six inches across at the widest point. The velvety leaves are similar to mullein. They clasp the stem as they approach the top, becoming smaller as they go. The spindle-shaped, mucilaginous root is perennial. It is five to six inches long, an inch and a half at the thickest part, succulent, branching, brown, and aromatic.

Inula was well known to the Greeks and is said to have been named for Helen, wife of Menelaus, who was believed to have had an armful of the plant when Paris abducted her to Phrygia. Another explanation of the name is that the best plants grew on the island of Helena. Before Linnaeus, however, the plant was known as *Enula campana,* as it grew wild in Campania.

Julius Augustus, said Pliny, ate *Inula* roots every day to aid digestion "and cause mirth." Galen proclaimed it "good for the passions of the hucklebone called sciatica." In Anglo-Saxon medicine, elecampane was used in England before the Norman conquest. The Welsh physicians of the thirteenth century called it "marchala."

Medieval herb and monastery gardens all cultivated elecampane. The plant contains an active, bitter principle called helenin, inulin, acrid resin, volatile oil, inulenin, and mucilage, among others. The active ingredient, helenin, is used as an antiseptic in pulmonary diseases. It is contained in many proprietary medicines. Inulin, from the root of elecampane, undergoes hydrolysis to a form of fructose, which is used in diabetic bread. The roots of dahlias and Jerusalem artichokes are similar.

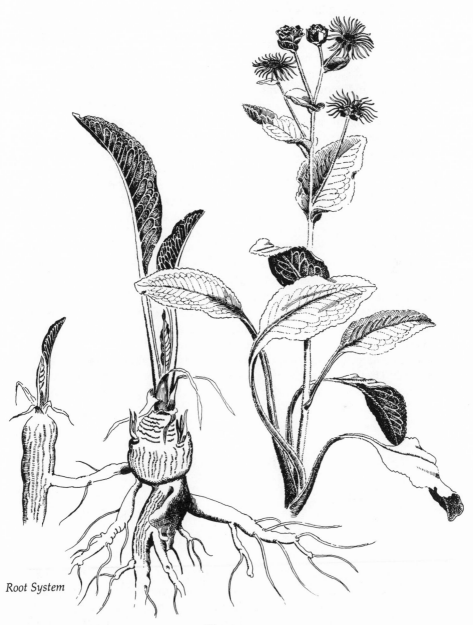

Root System

Elecampane

Present-day herbalists use the root of elecampane as a tonic for pulmonary complaints and for coughs. It is a safe and efficient home medicine for bronchitis and asthma. The dose is one teaspoonful of the decoction taken three times a day. As an embrocation, it may be used externally in the treatment of sciatica and neuralgia. The distilled water of the herb and root will remove blemishes from the skin.

The medicinal action of elecampane is diuretic, antibiotic, tonic, antiseptic, astringent, and gentle stimulant. Modern research has proved that the use of elecampane in the treatment of pulmonary diseases has a solid basis. Its active, bitter principle, helenin, is a powerful antiseptic and bactericide. One part to ten thousand makes a solution that will kill any ordinary bacterial organisms by the use of a few drops of it. In Spain, it is being used successfully as a surgical dressing.

We know that elecampane was used by the early frontier doctors in the United States. Robert D. Foster, a botanic "Indian" doctor, wrote a book containing 204 "receipts." In the 25th he listed elecampane, among other plants, as a cure for croup. The plant was observed in New York State in 1875 by John Burroughs, who wrote, "One may see a large slice taken from a field by elecampane. . . ."

As a garden plant, elecampane will grow readily from seed if sowed in a spot where it can receive plenty of water, but in which drainage is good. The roots may be started in a cold frame with soil that is a mixture of sand and loam. Dipping the root section in rotane insures rapid growth. The bright, showy, yellow flowers are an added reason for having this useful medicinal plant available in the garden.

ST. JOHN'S-WORT

ST. JOHN'S-WORT *Hypericum perforatum* L.
HYPERICACEAE

St. John's-wort is a hardy perennial found in uncultivated ground, meadows, and roadsides. The stems are branching, the leaves opposite, pale green, sessile, oblong with pellucid spots of oil glands which can be seen if the leaf is held up to the light. Bright yellow flowers grow in terminal cymes.

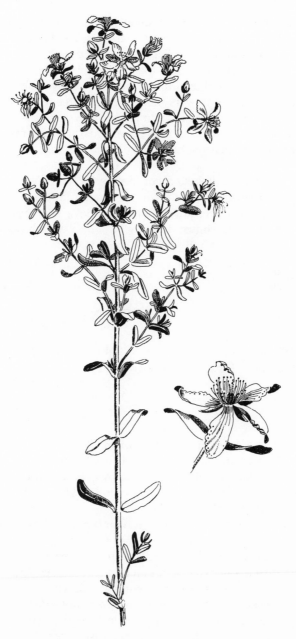

St. John's-wort

Medically, St. John's-wort is aromatic, astringent, expectorant, nervine, and vulnerary. It is used in pulmonary disease, bladder trouble, diarrhea, jaundice, and nervous depression. Because of its nervine properties, it can be used for insomnia and to prevent bedwetting.

Externally it is used as a fomentation to relieve caked breasts.

Oil made from the flowers that have been steeped in a jar with olive oil and allowed to stay in the sun for a few weeks to a month or more, is strained and used to treat bruises, wounds, and skin problems. If kept in a dark-colored glass bottle in a cool place it will keep for a year or more.

There are many folk beliefs concerning St. John's-wort. One is that if sprays are hung in the window on the twenty-fourth of June, St. John's birthday, they will keep away "ghosts, devils, and thunderbolts." On the twenty-ninth of August, the day St. John was beheaded, the leaves are supposed to show red spots.

VALERIAN

VALERIAN *Valeriana officinalis* L.
("SETWALL," "GARDEN HELIOTROPE")

VALERIANACEAE

Valerian is a true dual-purpose plant. Its flower is showy and fragrant in the garden, its root has been used for centuries as a cure for nervous disorders. Its virtues were known to the Anglo-Saxon leeches of the fifteenth century, and were extolled by the physicians of the medical school of Salerno in the ninth.

The plant grows to four feet tall with bipinnate foliage and fragrant pink-to-lavender flowers that appear in flat, terminal clusters. The rootstock, which is the part used medicinally, is short and up to three quarters of an inch in diameter. It has an unpleasant odor said to account for the name "Phu," by which the plant was known to the ancients.

Valerian is an anodyne, an antispasmodic, and a non-narcotic nervine.

A standard infusion of fresh rootstock, two teaspoons to one pint boiling water, taken cold, a small wineglassful three times a day half an

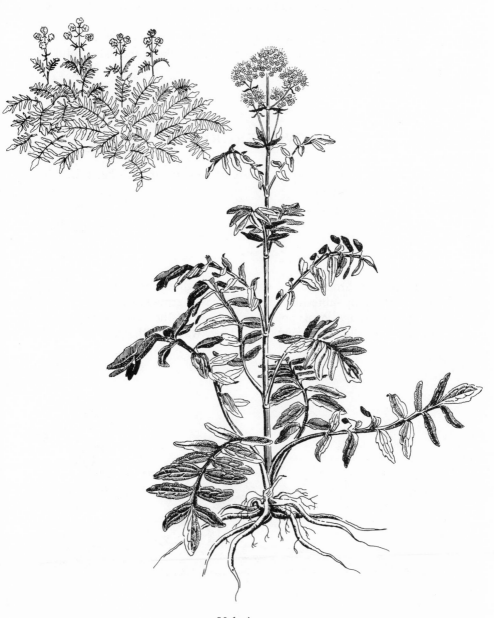

Valerian

hour before meals, is a good treatment for nervousness or nerve-caused diseases.

An extract prepared by soaking two teaspoonsful of rootstock in water for twenty-four hours, then strained, may be taken, one-half cupful, at bedtime.

WINTERGREEN

WINTERGREEN
("PARTRIDGEBERRY,"
"CHECKERBERRY")

Gaultheria procumbens L.

ERICACEAE

The plant is aromatic and smooth throughout. Branches grow erect from creeping or subterranean stems. Leaves grow mostly in clusters at the ends of stems, oval, oblong, narrowed at the base, short-petioled with margins slightly revolute (rolled backward), with very low, bristle-

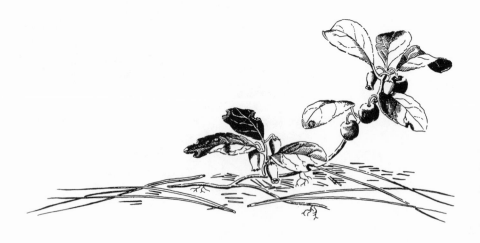

Wintergreen

topped teeth. The top side of the leaf is dark green and shiny, the underside is pale. Flowers grow in the axils. They are usually solitary, but occasionally two grow together. The fruit is bright red and five lobed.

Principal constituents of wintergreen are methyl salicylate, triacontane (a paraffin), an aldehyde, an alcohol, and an ester. It is a stimulant, diuretic, rubefacient, antirheumatic, carminative, anodyne, tonic, and emmenagogue.

An infusion of the leaves (standard brew) may be taken internally as a tea or used as a hot compress for headache, rheumatic pains, sciatica, or pains in the joints or muscles.

An infusion may also be used as a gargle for sore throat or as a douche for leucorrhoea.

YARROW

YARROW
("MILFOIL")

Achillea millefolium L.

COMPOSITAE

Authorities differ as to whether yarrow is native or naturalized to North America. If the latter be true, certainly yarrow is no johnny-come-lately, because reports from the year 1724 tell us of its use as a vulnerary by the Illinois and Miami Indian tribes.

Its botanic name derives from Achilles of Homeric fame, who is said to have cured his soldiers' wounds with yarrow. A more fanciful version tells that the infant Achilles was dipped into a bath of yarrow by his mother, who held him by his heel. This accounted for his invulnerability to wounds, except for his heel.

Yarrow is astringent, tonic, vulnerary, stimulant, diaphoretic, alterative, and emmenagogic. It contains an aromatic volatile oil, achellein, achilleic acid, resin, tannin, gum, and earthy ash. The whole herb is used medically by herbalists today. It dilates the pores, producing copious sweating, and is a valuable aid in reducing fevers and ridding the body of impurities. It may be used as a quinine substitute.

A strong infusion (double standard brew) is excellent for cleansing open wounds and preventing infection. It contracts mucous membranes

211

and blood vessels and is useful to stop hemorrhages. A poultice of bruised fresh leaves and flowers is soothing to rashes, and an infusion of the flowers is recommended for relief from acne.

Taken internally, yarrow is excellent for colds and fevers and the discomforts caused by them: headaches and muscular pains.

A gargle, made as a standard infusion, is a relief for sore throat.

The crushed fresh blossoms worked into lard, oil, or cold cream make

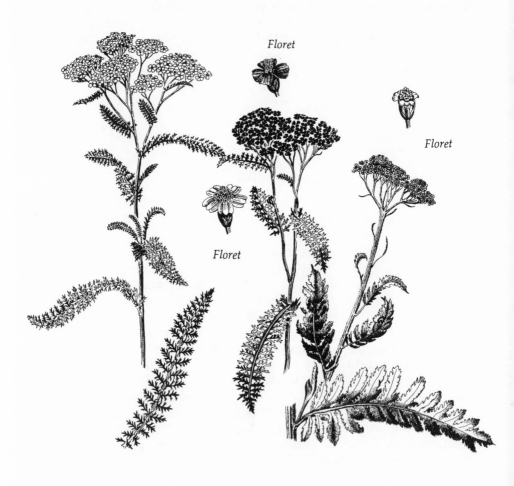

Floret

Floret

Floret

Yarrow

a salve that is useful in treating skin irritations and the itching of dry scabs on healed cuts. A standard decoction taken cold before meals, a wineglassful at a time, over a period of several weeks or more, is a good general tonic, helpful after an illness or period of stress. The decoction can be combined with any homemade wine and can be kept in the refrigerator for several months.

The Micmac Indians of Canada used yarrow as a sweat bath to cure colds, and we use the blossoms in a hot bath, preceded and followed by drinking a cup of the hot infusion.

The light-green, feathery leaves of yarrow, topped with pearly-white terminal cymes, made up of many tiny, white, daisy-like florets, are a common sight in the countryside. In our gardens we can add red and mustard-yellow flowering varieties to beds of the common white. All of these have the same properties and do well in any sunny location and any type of soil. The availability of yarrow makes it a boon to our good health, a plant to use and enjoy, to cut on a summer day when the Moon, under whose protection it grows, is on the increase.

In ancient China, fifty yarrow stalks were used to consult the oracle, *I Ching, The Book of Changes.* One stalk was put aside, and the remaining forty-nine divided, at random, into two heaps. From this point on, a complicated procedure was used to arrive at a hexagram and its interpretation.

The new-laid garden . . .
Rocks settling in harmony
In soft winter rain

SHADO

My very bone-ends
Make contact with the icy quilts
Of deep December

BUSON

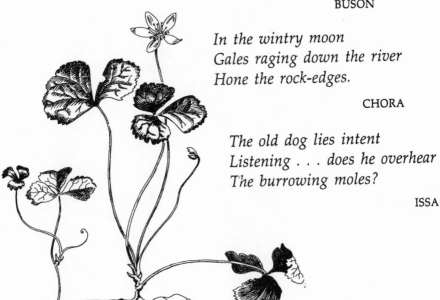

In the wintry moon
Gales raging down the river
Hone the rock-edges.

CHORA

The old dog lies intent
Listening . . . does he overhear
The burrowing moles?

ISSA

IX

Winter:
Season of Tisanes

The snow, crystal white, unmelted since Thanksgiving, glistens under moonlight. Polaris is high in the bright heaven, eleven hundred years from its eventual peregrination up the northern sky to cede its place to Vega as polestar. Eleven hundred years, a drop of water in the sea, a grain of sand in the desert compared to the years stretching back to prehistory, a time when Saturn, god of sowing and husbandry, lived on earth as a just and benevolent king of Italy. Saturn, who taught the people to till the soil and live in peace with each other, whose reign is believed to be the fabled Golden Age when war and love of money were unknown, when there was neither slavery nor private property, and all people shared alike the earth's bounty.

215

The Saturnalia, which reenacted the genial innocence of the good monarch's reign, was celebrated in ancient Rome for seven days and seven nights, from the seventeenth to the twenty-third of December. Master and slave changed places during this festival of mirth and good will, prince and pauper were equal, gifts were bestowed lavishly, and to ask was to receive.

Does our exchange of gifts at Christmas derive from this ancient source? Winter is a good time to do some research, but now our kettle is boiling, and we must choose some herbs to make tea for guests who will be arriving soon: comfrey, raspberry leaves, elder flowers, wintergreen, a few cloves, and curls of dried orange peel. This tisane, or infusion of herbs, sweetened very lightly with natural honey, tastes so good that it is like gilding the lily to say that it also contains iron, magnesium, potassium, peptic acid, and phosphorus, is anti-bacterial, and stimulates hydrochloric acid in the stomach.

Winter is a season that is hard on our bodies; keeping warm takes a great deal of energy that in other seasons is released for specific body functions. Heat and energy are interchangeable. When energy is being used for heat it is necessary for us to drink teas that will compensate for the loss of energy in other areas.

There are teas to warm us when we come in from the cold. Try combining:

One part chamomile
One part costmary
Two parts red clover
Two parts stinging nettle
Two parts thyme
A grating of fresh ginger and whole nutmeg

As you increase your supply of dried herbs, you will experiment with different combinations and flavors. Here are a few suggestions to start with, good winter teas for warmth and sociability.

Two parts marjoram and thyme
One part apple mint and hyssop

Two parts lemon balm (melissa) and comfrey
One part sage

Two parts chamomile
One part red clover and anise seeds

216

Two parts comfrey
One part each lavender, spearmint, and sage

Many teas taste pleasant, yet have specific medicinal uses too.

For High Blood Pressure:
Chopping wood and shoveling snow sometimes raise blood pressure.
Equal parts of parsley (leaves and root), anise, chamomile, and fenugreek

To Purify the Blood:
This is important at the beginning and end of winter.
Two parts burdock root and comfrey
One part each wormwood, nettle, peppermint
Two parts primrose (leaves and flowers) and sage
One part each dandelion root, yarrow, and a few whole cloves
Equal parts raspberry and violet leaves, red clover, coriander

Healing and Soothing Teas for Bronchitis:
Equal parts ground ivy, elecampane root, eucalyptus leaves, and mallow root
Two parts comfrey and fenugreek
One part each anise seeds, witch grass rhizomes
Equal parts mullein, horehound, lungwort, and thyme
Equal parts coltsfoot, mullein, comfrey, mallow root

For Flatulence or Digestive Discomfort:
Equal parts chamomile, peppermint, lemon grass, anise, and a little dried
    orange, lemon, or grapefruit rind
Equal parts lemon balm (melissa), catnip, caraway seeds, and fennel seeds

For Chest and Lung Congestion:
One part boneset, one part yarrow
Two parts mullein, two parts eucalyptus
Two parts coltsfoot, two parts comfrey
One part each plantain, primrose flowers, nettle

To Increase the Flow of Bile, to Relieve Gall-Bladder Condition:
Two parts each parsley and stinging nettle
One part each yarrow, burdock root, and peppermint

217

For Colic:
Chamomile or catnip; for young babies, one tablespoon at a time of the warm infusion

For a Mild Laxative:
Two parts chickweed
One part each hyssop, yarrow, fenugreek, caraway, and fennel

For a Cough:
Two parts each coltsfoot and horehound
One part anise

Equal parts elecampane root, lungwort, and a few juniper berries

Two parts comfrey, two parts dill

One part marjoram and anise

To Soothe the Nerves:
Equal parts chamomile, blue vervain, anise

Equal parts borage, lavender, lemon balm

For Influenza:
Equal parts boneset, comfrey, coltsfoot

One part catnip, a tablespoon natural honey and lemon peel

Two parts plantain, St. John's-wort, comfrey
One part boneset, catnip, and one tablespoon honey

For Insomnia:
Everyone needs more hours of sleep in winter, so if you have trouble getting to sleep, take one of these harmless and helpful teas.

One part blue vervain, primrose flowers
Two parts chamomile

Equal parts agrimony, lavender, fennel seeds

Equal parts catnip, blue vervain, anise

Equal parts agrimony, chamomile, dill

For Hoarseness:
One part mullein, coltsfoot, stinging nettle
One or two tablespoons natural honey

Two parts each mallow flowers and root, salad burnet

For the Liver:
This is important for non-vegetarians.

One part dandelion root
Two parts peppermint, anise
One part dandelion root
Two parts sweet woodruff, rosemary

For Menstrual Cramps:
In winter, exposure to cold at the time of menstruation often causes cramps.

Equal parts raspberry leaves, lady's mantle

Equal parts meadowsweet, rosemary

Two parts St. John's-wort

One part tansy (tansy should not be taken by pregnant women, substitute sweet cicely)

For Stomach Ulcers:
Comfrey, calendula, fenugreek, equal parts
Stinging nettle, ground ivy, slippery elm, equal parts

For a Tonic:
Meadowsweet, bearberry, thyme, equal parts
Lemon balm (melissa), basil, raspberry leaves, equal parts

For Urinary Trouble:
Two parts parsley root
One part horsetail, sage, and a few juniper berries

For Cystitis:
Two parts corn silk
One part lovage root and meadowsweet
Equal parts bearberry, parsley seed, rose hips

In all teas except those for insomnia or stomach ulcers, the following additions may be made for flavor: a few cloves, a sprinkle of cinnamon or allspice, a drop or two of almond extract.

A special tea for acne is made by using burdock and comfrey root, anise, and fennel seeds in a decoction. Drink three to four cups a day, unsweetened.

Acne is also helped by holding the face over a pot of water in which comfrey leaves, violet leaves, purslane leaves, anise, and fennel seeds are simmering.

The provident winter kitchen will have two herb shelves, one which we call the medicine shelf, and the other the condiment shelf. Many excellent foods will borrow from the medicine shelf, so the division is not absolute—perhaps a seasonal obsession with order, however artificial.

THE MEDICINE SHELF

agrimony	elder flower
bearberry	eucalyptus
boneset	garlic
burdock root	ground ivy
burnet (*Sanguisorba minor*)	horehound
cayenne	horsetail
chamomile	lady's mantle
clover (*Trifolium pratense*)	meadowsweet
coltsfoot	mullein
comfrey	raspberry leaves
dandelion root	vervain
elecampane	yarrow

THE CONDIMENT SHELF

allspice	fenugreek
anise	ginger
basil	marjoram
cinnamon	mint
cloves	sage
coriander	wintergreen
dried orange, lemon peel	

While we have these lists before us, it is a good time to talk about the gentle art of compounding herbal teas and remedies. From the seventy-odd herbs in this book, you may use twenty or so the first year you begin using herbs to preserve health and remedy imbalances. Perhaps you will approach the whole matter slowly and decide to start with ten, get to know them completely by sight, touch, taste, smell, history, constituents, and medical action. Perhaps you are already quite expert in this. In any case, there is a useful rule of thumb in combining herbs. It is based on the triangle. If you use three herbs together, one, the apex of the triangle, will be strong. Two, the angles at the base of the triangle, will be mild. Or all three will be of equal, mild strength. Example:

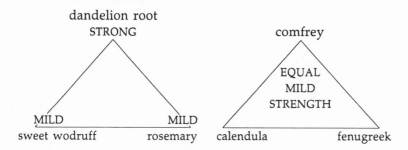

When we use "strong" in an herbal formula, we may mean that one herb, the one we place at the apex of the triangle, is a specific for the condition. The other two may aid this herb to do its job. Many herbal teas have five, six, or even more ingredients. Let us look at a tea which is used to warm a person after being exposed to cold:

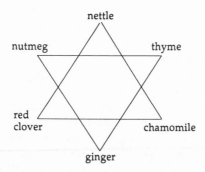

The basic triangle has nettle at the apex with two "helpers," red clover and chamomile, at the base. Nutmeg, ginger, and thyme comprise the second triangle, all of which add to the warming abilities of nettle.

221

Experience with herbs will develop a psychic rapport. You will know, without working it out consciously, what is needed. Should you decide on a specific curative herb but be somewhat indecisive about the helpers, it is sometimes helpful to use a pendulum. First, place the herbs that you find hard to choose between on a table and hold a pendulum over them, one at a time. Ask your pendulum in each case, "Is this the correct herb to put in this mixture?" The pendulum will give the affirmative answer if it is appropriate, a negative answer if the herb is not a good choice. For those who have not used a pendulum before, this is the way it works. When you first get your pendulum, ask it, "If the answer to a question I ask you is affirmative, which way will you swing?" After you receive the answer, then ask, "If the answer to my question is negative, which way will you move?" The way your pendulum responds this first time will be the way you should henceforth interpret it.

In winter, when the living essence of an herb returns to the root to conserve energy for the summer, so do we seem to gather in our resources and store our strength. Dreaming, remembering, projecting into the future, we enjoy a season of inner growth and preparation. Something occurs to us as, in reverie, we see our summer herb garden. Why should we be tied to straight lines and squares? Some changes will be made this year. There is power in a circle: the Sun, invincible, is a disc; the Moon at its brightest is round; the halo effect in the sky is circular. With our magic marker, on a large pad, we draw a circle. Four herbs ruled by the Sun will share this inner circle: marigolds, chamomile, salad burnet, and rosemary. In the very center there will be a statue of St. Fiacre, patron saint of gardeners. Born in Ireland before 600 A.D., Fiacre sought a solitary life in France where St. Faron, Bishop of Meaux, gave him land near Brie. There Fiacre built a hermitage and planted and tended a garden of herbs and vegetables which he used to cure the sick and feed the poor. The good saint's birthday is still celebrated on August thirtieth. French carriages called "fiacres" were used by Parisians who drove the seventeen miles from Paris to Meaux to worship at his shrine.

The triangles will be planted in rows of four, three, two, and one plants, to give them the power of Pythagoras' triangle, which he called the Holy Tetractys. One plus two plus three plus four equals ten, which he considered the perfect number. These triangular beds may be used for orange, apple, peppermint, spearmint. This will keep the varieties apart, a good precaution as mints cross-pollinate with the greatest of ease. At the apex of each triangle we may choose an accent of tall southernwood, tansy, sweet cicely, angelica.

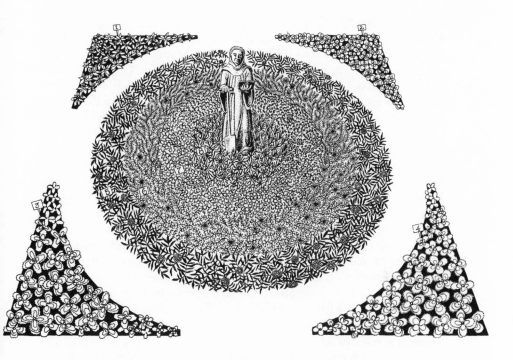

The herb garden: (1) English peppermint; (2) orange mint; (3) spear-mint; (4) apple mint; (5) dwarf marigold; (6) chamomile; (7) salad burnet; (8) rosemary; with St. Fiacre in the center.

After we have made these dream diagrams for our next summer's garden, we consult our seed catalogues. This is a satisfying event, a self-actualization that gives reality to our dream. But as we finish writing our known needs for next spring, our eye strays down the page to caraway-scented thyme, creeping woolly yarrow (very rare, says the catalogue), Vatican dwarf sage, golden spearmint. Should this heady list be mailed in the ordinary way, put in the post office, sent on its flight with a first-class stamp? Or should it, like the letters we wrote to Santa Claus as a child, be burned on the hearth, its essence wafted up the chimney in magical smoke?

As Christmas approaches we remember an Irish fairy tale, retold many times, about a little boy who believed in fairies and shared his milk and porridge with them by leaving a little saucer on the hearth each night. When his mother fell incurably ill, the Little Folk helped him to find the Seven Precious Herbs: chamomile, pennyroyal, self-heal, rue, tansy, yarrow, and thyme. Before the cock crowed on Christmas morning, he brewed a tea for his mother who then recovered.

A good introduction to herbs for young people is to help them make little bags, each of a different color, that can be filled with the seven precious herbs, tied with ribbon, and hung on the Christmas tree to be presented to visiting friends.

January in snow country is a month of clear, cold days and long nights. We use or herb shelves lavishly; our root cellars and freezers seem inexhaustible with last summer's bounty. Like the old alchemists, we seek our mystical center. In early morning, insulated by silent snowfall, we search for all that is "incomprehensible, invisible, immeasurable, infinite. . . ."[1]

By February's end, there are empty space on our herb shelf—how could we have used so much yarrow?—and will we never learn to dry enough peppermint? Frozen pumpkin for one more pie, enough basil for pesto and a last weekend of careful preparation. How the wood pile has dwindled! And the porch thermometer reading is thirty-nine degrees below zero. Must we listen to our household's favorite stories again . . . and again?

Where is that peaceful enjoyment of reading and writing letters that we felt last week? We should remember, but never do, that our problem is seasonal—cabin fever.

Primitive people believe that if you know the name of something, you have power over it. We agree. Cabin fever, we repeat, as we make a cup of melissa tea.

February twentieth; a duck on Herringbrook Road just laid four eggs. Ducks have built-in timers that can never be fooled; the omen is clear. In four weeks, when the ducklings hatch, it will be spring. Right on the cosmic calendar, the spring equinox falls on March twenty-first.

We have come through the unfailing progression of the seasons, from dandelion to duck, each feeling the ancient, inexorable urge for renewal at the appointed time. May we too learn to obey our inner wisdom, remembering, as we surround ourselves with healing herbs, that melissa (lemon balm) was known in ancient medicine as a remedy for melancholia, an herb to purge the body of all impurities and a means of inducing happiness.

[1] Gerard Dorn, "Physician Genesis," 1659.

CHICKWEED

CHICKWEED   *Stellaria media* L.
                                             CARYOPHYLLACEAE

Chickweed grows throughout the world and might almost be called an extension of man, as it can be found wherever he has made a home. Culpepper described it poetically as "a fine soft pleasing herb under the dominion of the Moon." Its action is demulcent, laxative, and refrigerant. Paracelsus called it the "elixer of life."

Chickweed is useful as an ointment and as an ingredient in embrocations that are used as wet applications or poultices. The plant is perfectly harmless and so can be used in varying proportions. As a mild cure for constipation, it can be taken three times a day, or in extreme cases every few hours until the bowels move normally. Put a handful of the fresh, or two tablespoons of the dried, herb in a quart of water and boil until half the liquid has evaporated. Drink warm, a cupful at a time.

Stiff neck, back, or joints, or bursitis can be helpfully treated by a poultice made of the following:

Mix equal parts of chickweed, cabbage leaves, leaves and flowers of thyme, one teaspoon cayenne pepper blended with powdered slippery elm and fenugreek. Moisten with hot cider vinegar until the mixture has the desired consistency. Spread on a cloth and apply warm. Cover the poultice with a piece of plastic for longer retention of heat.

The above ingredients, steeped overnight in water that has been brought to a boil, may be used as wet applications or in a hand or foot bath. This formula can be kept several days in a cool place, and warmed again as used. Do not boil again.

Chickweed, like dandelion, purslane, and pigweed, makes a healthy and delicious salad or cooked green. It is rich in copper and iron.

An infusion (standard brew) of chickweed is soothing for stomach ulcers and digestive problems. The bruised fresh leaves are healing to skin irritation and insect stings.

Stellaria media is a long, vine-like, procumbent, annual plant, the egg-shaped leaves having short, sharp points that grow in pairs on the smooth, pale-green stem. Tiny, white, star-shaped flowers grow singly from axils of the leaves, or from terminal cymes. A toothed capsule

225

contains the seeds which are widely dispersed by the wind when they are ripe, as are the seeds of many common annuals and biennials. These seeds are well liked by canaries and are said to improve the quality of their voices. This I cannot attest to—I am tone deaf.

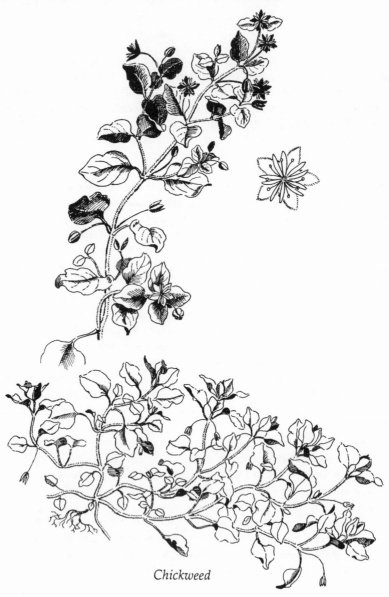

Chickweed

CONEFLOWER

PURPLE CONEFLOWER
("BLACK SAMPSON")

Echinacea angustifolia
D.C. Moench.
COMPOSITAE

The purple coneflower *E. angustifolia* is native to North America and grows west of Ohio and on the prairies. The stem is one to two feet high, the leaves lanceolate, hirsute, and narrowed at the tip and stem

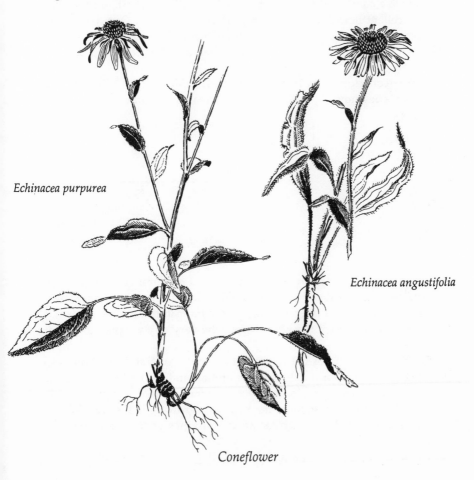

Echinacea purpurea

Echinacea angustifolia

Coneflower

ends. The root and rhizomes, the parts used medicinally, are tapering, cylindrical, slightly spiral, with a faint aromatic smell and a sweet taste which leaves a tingling sensation in the mouth. It is a hardy perennial with purple ray flowers and a bristly head.

Echinacea is used in the treatment of boils, erysipelas, gangrene, septicemia, cancer, and all blood impurities. It is useful in typhoid care, fevers, and fermentative dyspepsia. It is used today as an immune system stimulant. A tincture of *Echinacea* can be taken, five to ten drops a day, for a long time (for example, during the winter months) as an infection preventive. If an infection has already been contracted, twenty drops twice a day for a ten-day period is recommended.

Echinacea combined in equal parts with mullein, myrrh, and saffron is an excellent home cure for a streptococcus infection. One-half cup of the decoction can be taken hot, an hour before breakfast and between meals. Keep up the treatment for one week after the infection has disappeared.

Purple coneflower (*Echinacea purpurea* [L.] Moench) can be obtained from nurseries now. It does well and increases in home gardens.

CORN

CORN	*Zea mays* L.
	GRAMINACEAE

We usually think of corn as a delicious end-of-summer treat, perhaps roasted in its green sheath at a Labor Day picnic. If it grows in our own garden, we worry lest the raccoons, whose built-in timing mechanism is hard to beat, harvest it the night before the very day we plan to gather the ears.

Besides being one of the healthiest natural foods and the American Indians' great contribution to the diet of mankind throughout the tropic and temperate zones, corn is a valuable and inexpensive medicine, whose worth few would contest. Since its discovery, growing in the New World, it has been in constant use by shamans, frontier doctors, and modern pharmacologists.

The Indians of both Americas were well aware of its medicinal value.

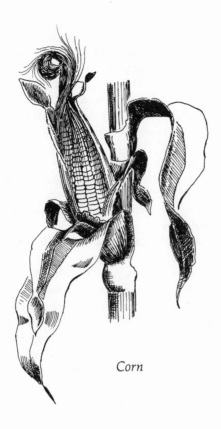

Corn

In the sixteenth century, Garcilaso de la Vega wrote in his *Royal Commentaries* that corn was "of great benefit in the treatment of affections of the kidney and bladder, among which are calculus and retention of urine." He went on to say that Spaniards were troubled with these problems, but that Indians, who ate corn and drank a beverage made from it, were not afflicted.

The Badianus Manuscript prescribed a decoction of ground corn for dysentery and to increase lactation in women. (Young mothers take note.)

Lloyd[1] tells us that domestic medicine in pioneer days used corn-silk tea for acute bladder infections.

[1] John Uri Lloyd, *Eclectic Medical Journal.* Sept. 1935 reprint from *Journal* of Sept. 1908, "Concerning Indian Medication."

229

Herbalists today know that corn silk is diuretic, lithostyptic, demulcent, antiseptic, and anodyne. Corn contains starch, sugar, fat, salts, water, yellow oil, maizenic acid, azotized matter, gluten, dextrine, glucose, cellulose, silica, phosphates of lime and magnesium, soluble salts of potassa (potassium hydroxide), and soda.

Corn silk, fresh or dried, contains maizenic acid, fixed oil, resin, chlorophyll, sugar-gum extractive, albuminoids, phlobaphine salt, cellulose, and water.

Vermont's well-known folk medicine advocate, the late Dr. D. C. Jarvis, recommended corn silk for hay fever, migraine, and asthma. The rationale of this suggestion is that the acids in corn shift the body chemistry from alkaline to acid. He recommended a tablespoon of the oil be taken at breakfast and dinner.

Modern herbalists use corn silk for bladder infections and for both chronic and acute cystitis, prostate problems, and bed-wetting.

A double-strength infusion (two ounces of corn silk to a pint of boiling water) can be taken every two or three hours, one to two teaspoons at a time, cold, on an empty stomach. Wait one-half hour before taking food.

One teaspoon of fresh silk or one-half teaspoon of the dried can be infused in one cup of boiling water for continuing treatment up to one week.

If you have access in the summer to fresh corn, grown in your own garden or bought from a local farmer, the silk can be eaten raw. Chop it fine, mix it into a bowl of yogurt with a teaspoon of molasses added and you will have a fine breakfast dish. Sprinkle a little wheat germ on top.

COSTMARY

COSTMARY
("BIBLELEAF,"
"ALEHOOF")

Balsamite major Desf
(*Chrysanthemumbalsamita*L.)

COMPOSITAE

Costmary is governed by Jupiter, the kindly, benevolent planet from whose name the word "jovial" is derived. Jupiter influences nutrition and cell building.

A native of the Orient, costmary is now found in almost every coun-

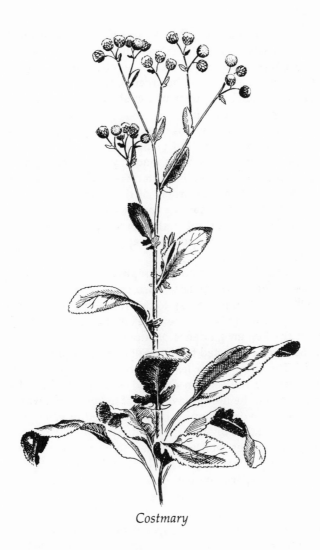

Costmary

try. It was brought to England in the early sixteenth century and to the United States by early English colonists. Its heyday of popularity occurred in the seventeenth century when Gerard said, "It groweth everywhere in gardens." In the twentieth century it has become rare in both English and American gardens.

Costmary is a hardy perennial which thrives in dry soil. Its oval, pale-green leaves are stiff and evenly but shallowly serrated. It grows two or three feet in height. When it flowers, usually August in New England, the blossoms are small, greenish-yellow, and unattractive; by the time this happens, the plant has a scraggly, unkempt appearance. It can be easily propagated from the creeping roots, so it is best to cut it back before it flowers. If grown in the shade, it sometimes does not flower and keeps a neat shape.

In the nineteenth century, costmary, combined with lavender, was popular as a scent for linens and blankets.

A slightly bitter medicinal tea is made by infusion. Allow it to steep only five minutes because of its bitter taste. *Green's Universal Herbal* (1532) recommends it for "disorders of the stomach and head." Other old books say that it "gives ease in gout, sciatica, and other like pains." For treatments of the latter, the herb should be steeped in olive or safflower oil for four days, strained, and applied locally. I have found it effective used in this way.

An Italian friend of mine said she snipped bits of fresh costmary leaf into scrambled eggs and omelets. I use this recipe frequently and am always delighted when guests try to determine the source of the pleasant "different" taste. This may be an example of costmary's nutritive value under the benign guidance of Jupiter.

When costmary emigrated to New England, it acquired a new name, "Bible leaf." The firm, tough leaves were used as place-marks in the Bible on Sunday; if the sermon dragged on interminably, the luckless parishioner chewed the minty-flavored leaf to keep him awake, much as we chew a mint-flavored gum to keep from nodding.

Costmary, which has digestive and antiseptic properties as well as its minty flavor, combines well with other herbs to make a healthy and aromatic tea for preventive as well as social use. Try some of these combinations and experiment with some of your own creative choosing.

One part costmary
One part vervaine
Two parts comfrey
One part lemon balm

One part costmary
Two parts comfrey
One part fennel seeds

One part costmary
One part comfrey
One part bugle
One part orange mint

One part costmary
Two parts chamomile
One part comfrey
One part anise seeds

FENUGREEK

FENUGREEK   *Trigonella foenum-graecum* L.
                         LEGUMINOSAE

In New England it is only in an exceptionally warm and long summer that fenugreek will flower and bear seeds before the first frost, but the powdered seeds are available from most health food stores and all botanical houses.

Fenugreek's major constituents include vitamins A and D, phosphates, lecithin, nucleoalbumin, riboflavin, niacin, pantothenic acid, choline, and

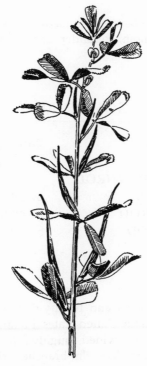

Fenugreek

iron in an organic form. It is mucilaginous, tonic, restorative, and sooth-ing. A poultice of mashed seeds soaked in dilute apple-cider vinegar is used for pains from gout, neuralgia, sciatica, swollen glands, and skin irritations. Its mucilaginous qualities make it a suitable vehicle for bind-ing together other medicinal herbs in poultices.

Irritations of the stomach and intestines are relieved by drinking a de-coction made by soaking one ounce of seeds in one pint of cold water for four hours, then allowing the mixture to boil for three minutes. The addi-tion of honey and a few drops of oil of anise, peppermint, or cloves will give a pleasant taste, and a cup of the tea may be taken three times a day.

In a diet for diabetics, the seeds may be sprouted and eaten on bread or in soups. Because of its similarity to the contents of cod liver oil, fenugreek has been used to treat rickets. It is also valuable in the diet of convalescents.

Commercially, fenugreek is used as a maple-sugar flavoring in con-fections and syrups.

Pulverized seeds can be used in making a curry powder along with seeds of cumin, cardamom, coriander, and turmeric.

GOLDENROD

TALL GOLDENROD	*Solidago altissima* L.
LATE GOLDENROD	*S. gigantea* L.
LANCE-LEAFED GOLDENROD	*S. graminifolia* L.
SWEET GOLDENROD	*S. odora* Ait.
CANADA GOLDENROD	*S. canadensis* L.
DOWNY GOLDENROD	*S. puberula* L.

COMPOSITAE

There are some hundred and twenty-five species of goldenrod of which sixty-five grow in the United States. Identification is not easy, but the various species can be divided roughly into five categories accord-ing to blossom form: plumelike, elm-branched, clublike, wandlike, and flat-topped. In all species the leaves are lanceolate, long sessile, smooth edged or slightly serrate, with only the veining differing from one spe-

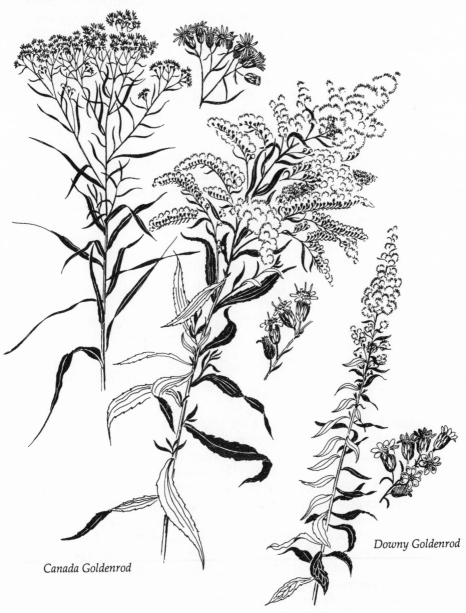

Lance-Leaved Goldenrod

Canada Goldenrod

Goldenrod

Downy Goldenrod

cies to another. In some the veins are parallel, some are feather veined.

Identification of the various species is not of great importance to the herbalist, as none are harmful. All species have the same medicinal properties: aromatic, astringent, diuretic, and vulnerary.

The whole herb, taken as an infusion, has a long history of being a remedy for kidney stones, flatulence, and vomiting. Externally it is used for wounds and as a hot compress to relieve headaches.

I have found it valuable, mixed with equal parts of red clover blossoms and elecampane, to prevent and relieve hay fever and similar respiratory allergies.

Make an infusion of the leaves and flowers of goldenrod and red clover blossoms, about a handful of each, fresh or dried, and add the liquid to an equal amount of elecampane root decoction. If a cup of this tea is taken every day for several weeks before the hay-fever season starts, it will prevent or lessen the allergic reaction.

GOLDTHREAD

GOLDTHREAD
("YELLOW ROOT,"
"CANKER ROOT")

Coptis groenlandica L.
(Oed.) Fern

RANUNCULACEAE

Goldthread grows in moist, cool woods. It is a small perennial with very long-petioled, evergreen leaves, one to two inches across, trifoliate, each segment broadly obovate, cuneiform (tapering to the base), with prominent veins. The leaves are shiny dark green above and paler beneath. In New England it blooms from May to July, with one, occasionally two, blossoms with five oblong, obtuse sepals and five small, club-like petals. The rhizomes, the part used, are threadlike and bright yellow.

Goldthread contains berberine, an alkaloid; albumin, a fixed oil, coloring matter, lignin, and sugar. It is bitter, digestive, stimulant, tonic.

A decoction of the root is useful to improve appetite and as a general stimulant to the entire system. It is also used as a mouthwash to heal sores in the mouth and as a gargle. As a tonic the dose is a tablespoonful three or four times a day, before each meal and in midafternoon.

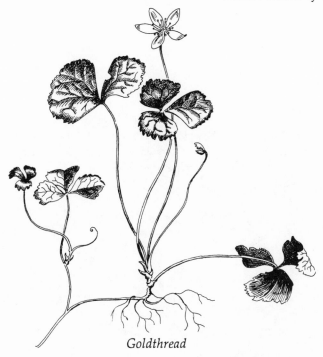

Goldthread

MYRRH

MYRRH   *Commiphora myrrha* (Nees.) Engl.
                                        BURSERACEAE

Myrrh is a shrub or small tree that grows in Arabia and northeast Africa. As a valuable and purifying incense it is usually thought of in connection with frankincense, in the Gospel of Matthew, II–11: "and when they had opened their treasures, they presented unto him gifts: gold, and frankincense and myrrh."

The part used is an oleo-gum-resin which is exuded when a cut is made in the bark.

As a medicine, myrrh is stimulant, healing, antiseptic.

A tincture is used in cases of inflamed sore throat or ulcers and as a

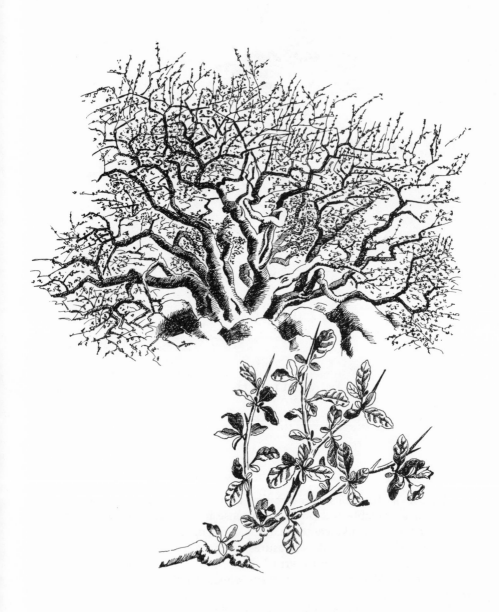

Myrrh

wash for ulcerated mouth and sore gums. Two to five drops at a time, in one-half glass water, can be taken as needed.

An infusion, one teaspoon of myrrh to one pint of boiling water, can be taken internally for bad breath or loose teeth. The dose is one teaspoonful four or five times a day.

It can be used in combination with purple coneflower and other herbs to treat streptococcus infection.

STRAWBERRY

STRAWBERRY	*Fragaria virginiana* L.
RASPBERRY	*Rubus idaeus* L.
	ROSACEAE

The strawberry, prized fruit of garden and refrigerator, is a perennial herb, one of twenty species of the genus *fragaria* of the rose family. A joy to northern gardens, the strawberry needs no winter protection other than the snow that falls so obligingly from November until April. The compound leaves have three leaflets; the white flowers grow in clusters at the end of a slender stalk. Varieties that produce few runners are best set in hills, prolific runner varieties in matted rows. Strawberries need a goodly supply of manure worked into the ground in the fall. The everbearing varieties have smaller fruit with fine flavor and are a boon to the busy gardener and herbalist.

William Coles, in *The Art of Simpling* (1656), advises, "Among strawberries sow here and there some Borage seed and you shall find the strawberries under those leaves farre more larger than their fellowes." Companionate planting was obviously well known in the seventeenth century, and this example still works like a charm. Not only are my berries "more larger" for their proximity to borage, but they have never been plagued by insects or disease.

The three-star gourmet rating of strawberries is equaled by the medicinal value of the leaves. Herbalists recommend them in cases of vomiting and diarrhea, for menstrual cramps, to prevent miscarriage, to increase milk during lactation, and for use before and after delivery. A standard infusion may be administered as often as needed, the strawberry being the mildest of the rose family. A tea can be given to infants who cannot tolerate any other food.

Raspberry is also a member of the rose family (*Rubus idaeus* is the European wild plant; there are American varieties). Raspberry leaves should be picked before the plant flowers for medicinal use. They are astringent, anti-mucreal (checks vaginal discharge), tonic, and stimulant. Malic and citric acids, pectin, calcium, and citrate of iron are all contained in the plant.

In a standard infusion the leaves are good for sore throat and ulcers of the mouth, and to reduce sudden high fever in children. Herbalists use it for eruptive diseases such as measles, chicken pox, and scarlet fever, also for nausea, as a healthy tea during pregnancy, and for intestinal influenza.

Strained and cooled, raspberry tea can be used as a douche for leucorrhoea. The fruit, like the strawberry, is a mild laxative.

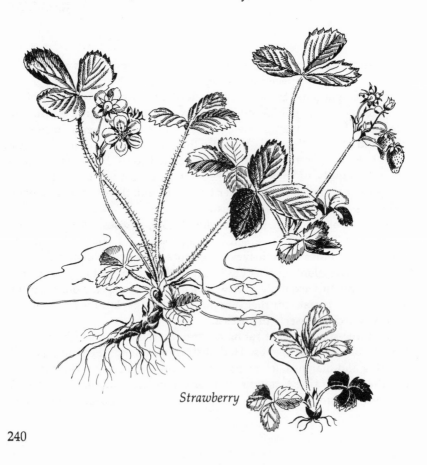

Strawberry

X

The Armchair Herbalist

An old friend who detested travel was a sought-after dinner guest because of his vast repertoire of stories that ranged from the caste system of the Mbaya in Brazil to the architectural eccentricities of the Pagoda of Six Harmonies in Hangchow. He had never been west of New Haven nor east of Nantucket, but in the book-strewn comfort of his study he roamed the world.

For those who will never plant a garden or collect a sprig of wild thyme, there is the option of becoming an armchair herbalist.

Herbal recipes turn up in unexpected places. Nicolai Gogol's character, the excellent housewife, Pulherya Ivanovna, distilled milfoil (yarrow) and sage with vodka to make a beverage that cured pain in the shoulder blades and loins. Vodka with peach stones, she asserted, would make a bump on the forehead disappear within a few minutes.

Pseudo Apuleius said, "Anyone have with him this herb (columbine)

. . . he will not be barked at by dogs." Had this bit of ancient wisdom been known to poor Mr. Gravely, who came once a month to read our electric meter, life would have been a happier affair for him. Our dog was a vociferous barker.

Odd medicinal advice knows no geographical boundaries; from England, China, Egypt, and America come some bizarre recommendations.

In Chaucerian England, John of Arden had a remedy for wounds called "Sanguis Veneris," which herbalist John Gerard described as "singular." The Honorable John's antidote was "to take of oile of olive a pint, the root alkanet two ounces, earth worms purged, in number twenty, boile them together and keep it to the aforesaid."

Another old English book recommends agrimony to be taken with "a mixture of powdered frogs and human blood" to cure all internal hemorrhages.

The Chinese, most of whose herbal medicine is valid today, had their foibles, too. Love philters were made from dragonflies. It was believed that if the dragonflies were buried in the house on the fifth day of the fifth month, the eyes would be transformed into blue pearls.

The Chinese used a contraceptive which is unlikely to regain popularity. Catch a scorpion, tear off all its legs, roast the body in ashes, smear glue on the wings of an autumn cicada, sprinkle the scorpion ashes on it, knead well and spread the resulting dough on the abdomen of the woman, three fingers below the navel. If, at some later date, she wants a child, the contraceptive can be undone if she swallows the saliva of a toad.

From an old family diary comes this early American liniment for sciatica made as follows: "In equal parts of olive oil and red wine boil: three puppy dogs, one pound earthworms, one handful each of rosemary, bay leaves, lavender, and thyme, yellow wax, and goose grease."

Another early American recommendation, this one for toothache, comes from no less a dignitary than the Reverend Cotton Mather: "Thrust the eye of a needle into the Bowels of a Sow Bug, and the matter which it fetches out, put in the hollow tooth, if it be such as aches." If that doesn't work, try the thigh bone of a toad applied to an aching tooth; it "rarely fails in easing the pain."

From the Ebers Papyrus of fifteen thousand B.C. come two recipes for the prevention of falling or thinning hair which are of interest to the armchair herbalist but might present some difficulties for the practitioner. The first calls for equal parts of the claw of a dog, decayed palm leaves, and the hoof of an ass, all boiled together and rubbed on the head. The second is a scalp lotion made from Khet plants, collyrium, gazelle dung, hippopotamus fat, and oil.

It is pleasant to reflect, as we sit comfortably before a fire, that some of the more domesticated herbs, common to every kitchen garden and chain-store spice shelf, have their moment of fame in song and legend.

> *Are you going to Scarborough Fair?*
> *Parsley, sage, rosemary, and thyme*
> *Remember me to one who lives there,*
> *She was once a true love of mine.*

Rosemary, *Rosmarinus officinalis*, is the gentle Cinderella of the "Ballad of the Rosemary." When Mary rode to Egypt with the baby Jesus, flowers along the way began their blossoming. "The lilac lifted up her proud and plumy branches, the lily spread her cup. Only the green rosemary, born petal-less and mild, grieved that it owned no benison of sweetness for the Child." Becoming weary, Mary rested beside a river; while the Baby slept, she washed His clothes. Where could she hang them? "The lily breaks beneath them, the lilac stands too tall." So she laid them on the rosemary who "held them all morning to the sun."

> *I thank you gentle rosemary.*
> *Henceforward you shall bear*
> *Blue clusters for remembrance*
> *Of this blue cloak I wear.*
>
> *And not your blossoms only,*
> *I give you as reward,*
> *But where his raiment clung to you*
> *Which clad the little Lord.*
>
> *All shall be aromatic,*
> *Said Mary, for I bless*
> *Leaf, stem, and flower*
> *That from this hour*
> *Shall smell of holiness.*

Mandrake, a more sinister herb than the gentle rosemary, was put to song by John Donne in the sixteenth century when he wrote:

> *Goe and catche a falling starre*
> *Get with child a mandrake roote*

But the history of the mandrake, *Atropa mandragora* (now called *Mandragora officinarum*), of the genus *Solanaceae*, goes back to 1375 B.C. It was cultivated in Egyptian gardens. Mandrake seeds were found in the tomb of Tutankhamen along with glazed faience representations of the fruit. Both Egyptians and Greeks knew the plant to be narcotic, anesthetic, anodyne, and aphrodisiac.

Ancient Greek herb gatherers believed that the mandrake should be cut while facing west and then only after three circles had been drawn around it with a sword. In medieval Europe, dogs were used to pull up the root, which grows three to four feet deep in the earth. A dog was chained to the plant and a piece of meat was placed a short distance in front of him. Because the mandrake root is often cleft, giving it the appearance of legs, it was thought to resemble a man and was said to emit a frightful scream when uprooted, which meant instant death to all who heard it. The dog, of course, dropped dead.

Mandrake roots of human form were much in demand for use as charms. When the true root became scarce and could not supply the market, byrony roots, somewhat sculpted, were substituted. In Germany these cosmeticized roots, called "Alraum," became minor works of art, some costumed as dolls. They were imported into England at the time of Henry VIII, and one of these may be seen today in the Wellcome Historical Medical Museum in London.

Fashion cooperates with the armchair herbalist today. After roughly a hundred years the pendulum has swung back to health and herbs as chic topics of conversation. In the late 1970's health food stores proliferated from Vasco Nuñez de Balboa's peaceful ocean to the cold gray shores of the Atlantic, stores with name such as "Nature's Own," "Narnia," "Eartherbs," "The Good Life," and "The Bean Bag." In 1873, Lydia Estes Pinkham sold her first bottle of Vegetable compound, a liquid guaranteed to restore to robust health any fragile female suffering the debilities of her sex and enable her to "do her own washing." It contained:

Jamaica dogwood (*Piscidia erythrina*)
Pleurisy root (*Asclepias tuberosa*)
Black cohosh (*Cimicifuga racemosa*)
Golden ragwort (*Senecio aureus*)
Licorice (*Glycyrrhiza*)
Dandelion (*Taraxacum officinale*)
Gentian (*Gentiana lutea*)

Vitamin B-1 (Thiamine hydrochloride)
Ethyl alcohol (used solely as a solvent and preservative)

This was an age when "vegetable" had a charisma beyond the garden patch, and "health" was a preoccupation that one-upped politics and equalled religion. Nineteenth-century food reformer, Sylvester Graham, persuaded students and faculty of the newly founded Oberlin College to eat graham bread (named after him) and drink burnt-toast coffee.

Graham was not the only nineteenth-century character to focus his attention on the problems of health. George Catlin, better known for his paintings of the American Plains Indians, wrote a slim and curious seventy-six page health book, *The breath of life and its effects upon the enjoyments and life of man. . . .*", published in New York in 1861 by J. Wiley.

On the title page Catlin proclaimed:

> *All life [on earth] is Breath*
> *All else [on earth] is Death.*

Artist Catlin spent many years living with Indian tribes in Central and South America as well as in the North American West. He was impressed with the way Indian mothers held their babies' mouths closed to establish nose rather than mouth breathing. "Air entering through the nose is as different when it reaches the lungs as distilled water is from water obtained from a frog pond" (or a city water purification plant—with all its chemicals!).

"The breath of Life was breathed into man's nostrils," said author Catlin, and should continue to "be breathed in the same manner."

This theory of breathing was subscribed to in the eighteenth century by the author of the *Critique of Pure Reason*. Immanuel Kant, one of the greatest figures in the history of philosophy, a frail and gentle man who lived beyond eighty, explained his theory when he was asked why he took his daily walks alone. If he took a companion along, he said, he would talk. If he talked, he would breathe through his mouth, which would make him prone to colds, coughs, and lung problems. Being a sensible as well as brilliant man, he walked alone, breathed through his nose, and lived fifteen years past the allotted three score and ten.

An herbal variation of the coals carried to Newcastle belongs in the back-pack of every armchair herbalist. Carrying ginseng to China was popular in America at the end of the eighteenth century when trade with China was brisk and the American species of the family *Araliaceae* had an eager and high-priced market. Hunting the wild plant became a profitable quest. Daniel Boone, an early ginseng hunter in Virginia, accumulated nearly fifteen tons on one expedition. In Vermont, the father of Joseph Smith (founder of the Church of Jesus Christ of the Latter-day Saints) did his hunting of ginseng around Williamstown, Vermont. Neither Boone nor Smith were fated to grow rich on ginseng, in spite of the fact that the Chinese were paying five dollars a pound. Boone's roots, carefully dried, fell into a river, and their value depreciated before he reached his wholesale market. Smith hired a ship and a captain to deliver his ginseng to a Chinese broker. The captain delivered the cargo and collected the money, but Smith never saw the seafaring fellow again.

An armchair herbalist in the mood for name-dropping might start with Paracelsus, a name sure to provoke controversy. "The salt of man's urine," he told his contemporaries, who considered him a pretty didactic fellow, "hath an excellent quality to cleanse. . . . Man's dung . . . hath very great virtues because it contains in it all the noble essence, i.e., food and drink."

An orchid-growing friend in Oaxaca used to appreciate nothing so much as a jar of urine; the nicest orchids, it seems, are not above responding to a good dose of uric acid. Even the cellophane-wrapped Western world cannot help but take an occasional tangential look at the fact that over half the world raises its foodstuff by dint of what is euphemistically called "night soil."

The following bit of exotica comes from Uganda where the Bahima people are plagued by deep-seated abscesses.

To cure this condition, they buy herbs from the local medicine man, rub them over the swelling, then bury the herbs under a well-frequented piece of ground. The first person who steps over the buried herbs, it is said, breaks out with boils, and the original sufferer is cured.

A similar story comes from darkest New Hampshire. A friend's mother reported that her mother cured warts by tying a string around a piece of salt pork and burying it during the dark of the moon. When the string rotted, the wart would drop off.

For those who failed to collect blue vervain and agrimony in August, it will be comforting to know that insomnia can be cured by memorizing the begats of an ancient family of Cos. Hippocrates, 460–377 B.C., was said to be descended from Asclepius, the legendary physician-god who was the son of Apollo and the nymph Coronis. Here are the family begats:

Asclepius begat Podalirus
Podalirus begat Sostratus
Sostratus begat Dardanus
Dardanus begat Crisamis
Crisamis begat Cleomytades
Cleomytades begat Theodorus
Theodorus begat Sostratus II
Sostratus II begat Theodorus II
Theodorus II begat Sostratus III
Sostratus III begat Nebrus
Nebrus begat Hippocrates I
Hippocrates I begat Heraclides
Heraclides begat Hippocrates II, called Hippocrates the Great

A soporific list, better than counting sheep. I have never stayed awake past Sostratus II, but a friend, a somewhat unreliable type, claims to have reached Nebrus.

Truth lurks in strange places waiting to be recognized. Cettwy, an ancient Celtic astrologer-philosopher-physician of Wales, propounded fifteen rules for a long and happy life. His third rule seems very sensible indeed. "Man," he advised, "should eat when hungry, drink when thirsty, and rest when tired."

After a lapse of centuries another nugget of truth may be mined from Hostetter's *United States Almanac* for the year 1882, calculated for Boston, Pittsburgh, and New Orleans. A statement is made that few would fault, in spite of the fact that it is embedded in a soft sell for Hostetter's Stomach Bitters, "Physical vigor is the main safeguard of health. It repels and fights off the morbid elements which superinduce disease."

There is no better exercise than planting an herb garden! May this year's armchair herbalist be next year's gardener.

XI

The History of Herbs

The Ebers Papyrus is the oldest written herbal known to exist, written about 1500 B.C. It is now in the University of Leipzig. It names more than one hundred and twenty-five plants with eight hundred and eleven prescriptions for salves, poultices, gargles, inhalations, enemas, suppositories, pills, liquid medicines, and directions for fumigation.

The Egyptians of fourth thousand years ago suffered from many of the same diseases as does modern man. Diagnoses and remedies in the Papyrus cover burns, colic, constipation, cardiac disease, catarrh, cystitis, glandular swelling, leukemia, tumors, eye and throat infections, and worms. Honey and oil are named as suitable vehicles in which to mix herbal remedies.

In those days, doctors made house calls. They also set a precedent for medical teams. When the "asu" (doctor) rode up to your door on a donkey, he was accompanied by an "ashipu" (exorcist) and a "baru" (seer). The established routine went like this: The ashipu recited incantations over the patient, the baru, watching for signs or omens, interpreted them to the asu, who then judiciously prepared the correct herbal medicine.

About two hundred and fifty years later, in Greece, Aesculapius of Cos, son of the god Apollo and the nymph Coronis, founded the first spa. (For details of this lineage, see page 247.) It was in Epidaurus, where mountain air and sea breezes helped cures based on baths, fasting, and herbal decoctions, and the therapeutic use of music, drama, and games.

Ruins of the baths, temples, and stadium are visited every year by thousands of tourists. Our guide pointed out a large stone slab on which were inscribed some of the famous cures utilizing four hundred herbs. Six hundred years later these were compiled by Thales of Miletus and Pythagoras of Samos. By the time Theophrastus inherited Aristotle's library and wrote *De Plantis*, five hundred herbs were known and listed.

The sanatorium of Epidaurus was duplicated in other parts of Greece. Resident physicians, called "Aesclepiadae," faithfully recorded all cases treated, symptoms, diagnoses, and results. The study of these medical fact sheets gave birth to the art of prognosis and the study of the natural history of disease. All of this paved the way during the next eight hundred years for Hippocrates, who has been called the "father of medicine." Some of his thoughtful advice, which can be read in his *Aphorisms*, would be pertinent for us to consider today. For example: "look to the country and to the season before deciding on treatment," "in every treatment of the body, whenever one begins to endure pain, it will be relived by rest," and "of natures, some are well adapted for summer and some for winter."

If we move on another two hundred and fifty years, we come to Mithridates VI, Eupator of Pontus. This ruler had an extensive herb garden where he and his court physician, Crateus, collected, planted and used herbs from all over the known world. Some medicinal plants used today, notably *Eupatorium perfoliatum,* or boneset, were named to commemorate this ruler.

By the first century A.D. Pedanius Dioscorides, a Greek physician attached to the Roman armies, collected a vast amount of material about plants, which he recorded in his *De Materia Medica.* Some of these plants still appear in the official pharmacopeias, although each year takes its toll as synthetic drugs replace them. (Whether the active ingredient is as beneficial when taken out of its natural context is open to question.) A cursory list of herbs mentioned by Dioscorides gives us the feeling that we are scanning a guest list of old friends. We find: anise, belladonna, chamomile, cardamom, cinnamon, colchicum, coriander, dill, gentian, ginger, juniper, lavender, linseed, licorice, marjoram, mallow, mustard, pepper, rhubarb, thyme, wormwood.

The seed-bed of European medicine was the Alexandrian School which was founded about 250 B.C. in Egypt and reached its zenith under the Ptolomies. Its herbalists and botanists settled along the Mediterranean and followed the caravan routes to Jerusalem and Damascus.

By the eighth century A.D., the Arabs, who had learned from the Jewish teachers schooled in Alexandria, were making translations of Dioscorides, Galen,[1] and Hippocrates. When they conquered Egypt, they began to compile dictionaries of the Coptic language spoken by those Egyptians who had become Christians through the teachings of St. Mark. By the middle of the fourteenth century the first bilingual herbal was produced by Ibn Kabr. In this is mentioned other old friends: parsley, rue, trillium, wake-robin, asphodel.

In the ninth century, a famous medical school was established in Salerno, on the south coast of Italy, at the entrance to the inlet of the Tyrrhenian Sea. Said to have been founded by a Latin, an Arab, a Jew, and a Greek, it became the focal point of all medical knowledge of the time. It contained a medical college and a sanatorium and health resort for all of Europe, including those returning from the Crusades.

Another famous medical school was in Montpellier, just inland from the curve made by the Gulf of Lyons on the south coast of France. Its most famous pupil was Ramon Lull, called "Dr. Illuminatissimus," mystic, philosopher, alchemist, and searcher for the Philosopher's Stone.

In the thirteenth century, two brilliant men were so far ahead of their time that their opinions were ignored for three hundred years. Roger Bacon, English philosopher and Franciscan monk, wrote acidulous criticisms of the prevalent conventional opinions of his day and called upon the Church to take the lead in subjecting the mass (I might say "mess") of translated knowledge about medicine to analytical scrutiny. His views were considered heretical and he was imprisoned instead of praised.

Fifty years before the "admirable doctor" Bacon expressed his unconventional views, Moses Maimonides was forthright in his attack on the fallacies and inaccuracies of the translations of Galen, whose work was looked upon as gospel. Maimonides was not put in jail for his opinions, but this was possibly because he wrote in Arabic, which few could read, and only very fragmentary Latin translations were available.

---

[1] Galen, 130–200 A.D. systematized all medical knowledge. He was the undisputed authority until 1600.

As an herbalist, Maimonides also recommended capers, peppers, and wormwood. Modern medicine today has "discovered" that green peppers are high in vitamin C and wormwood is recognized as a diuretic. Also recommended as effective diuretics were: celery, carrots, valerian, and wild ginger. Blackberry leaves, onions, and asparagus were good, he said, for gall and kidney stones.

Two men, one Italian, one Swiss, propounded a philosophy of healing which we may find interesting to contrast with the materialism of twentieth-century medicine.

Marsilio Ficino was born in Florence, the son of Cosimo de Medici's personal physician. A devout Christian at a time when Cosimo was hoping to bring neo-Platonism back, his ideal was St. Augustine. He said the highest act of charity was to help man to keep healthy in mind and body and that "medicine without heavenly grace is ineffective and even harmful." Paracelsus, born Philippus Aureolus Theophrastus Bombastus von Hohenheim six years before the death of Ficino, was also the son of a physician. He believed that through wise use of plants whose qualities corresponded to their ruling planets, a beneficial astral influence could be directed into the body which would neutralize disease. Certain plants under the influence of their ruling planets were specifically indicated for certain diseases. Because of the difficulty involved in selecting the right plant for the right disease, and under the correct planetary conditions, Paracelsus said that spiritual perception was essential for a dedicated physician. He thought there was a vital essence in all forms of life, which he called "mumia," and that the universe was a manifestation of this life force which acted through differentiated forms. In contrast to this opinion, physicians today regard the universe as an accumulation of forms which can be considered separately and treated without regard for a unifying life force.

Philosophically remote from Paracelsus, modern medicine gives him credit for his use of calomel (mercurous chloride) as a diuretic and fungicide. This remedy was forgotten after his death and rediscovered in 1885 by Jendrassik. Later, calomel was used in a proprietary medicine called "Guy's Hospital Pills," in which it was combined with squill and digitalis.

Because he saw the spark of life as one in men, animals, and plants, Paracelsus considered food an important factor in man's health and nature.

In the fifteenth century, herbals were still based on the belief that four elements, with their respective properties, were reflected in all living things. Each element had two correspondences: fire was hot and dry; earth, cold and dry; air, hot and moist; and water, cold and moist.

Each zodiacal sign was believed to be controlled by one of the elements. Pisces, for example, was a water sign. Marsilio Ficino's theory that each part of the body was ruled by a different sign and planet was incorporated into this body of belief.

Four keys to medical treatment were used: the astrological sign governing the part of the body, the planet which influenced the sign, the plants dominated by the sign, and the element with which it was associated. Hips, thighs, and liver were believed to be controlled by Sagittarius, which was under the rule of Jupiter and was an earth sign. The plants dominated by Jupiter, and thus chosen to relieve ailments of hips, thighs, and liver were: agrimony, balm, betony, borage, chervil, chestnut, cinquefoil, dandelion, houseleek, hyssop, red rose, sage, and thistle.

One of these Jupiterian herbs, dandelion *(Taraxacum officinale),* is used today in herbal medicine to treat diseases of the liver because of its high taraxacin content.

The first herbal in the Americas was the Badanius Manuscript, called the "Aztec Herbal," which was written in the sixteenth century in the Nahautl language of the Indians of Mexico, and translated into Latin and Spanish. The original manuscript was in the Vatican until it was returned by the Pope on his trip to Mexico in 1990. It contains an extensive materia medica of plants, trees, flowers, and herbs. Narcotics and analgesics were known and used during operations and for general relief of pain. The hand-painted illustrations gave color keys to the terrain in which each plant was found, in water, among rocks, or in open fields.

Bezoar stones, calcareous concretions found in the stomachs of birds and animals, were prescribed to cure poisonings, snake bites, and heart trouble, and to expel worms. They had been used in China, Egypt, and India, and during the seventeenth and eighteenth centuries were the vogue in Europe. Valued as remedies, charms, and jewels, they sold for such high prices (sometimes more than one thousand dollars) that the poor were forced to rent them by the day. Queen Elizabeth owned a large bezoar set in gold.

Belief in the curative power of these stones came to America with the early English settlers. Governor Endicott of Salem sent a bezoar and an alleged unicorn horn, along with an herbal remedy, to the elder Governor Winthrop when his wife suffered from what was called a "mother fit," or hysteria. The herbal remedy contained anise, mint, mugwort, roses, and violets.

Another import from the mother country was a belief in the Doctrine of Signatures, which taught that the same benign Providence that placed herbs on the earth also provided a clue, through their shape and color, to guide man in their proper curative use. Lungwort (*Pulmonaria officinalis*), a member of the borage family, has white spots on its leaves. This was thought reason enough to use it for those diseases causing spots on the lungs. Liverwort (*Anemone hepatica*), has liver-shaped leaves, thought to be a clue to its use in treating malfunctions of the liver. Both plants are still considered mildly healing.

Seventeenth- and eighteenth-century English herbals continued to be published and read with avidity. Turner, Greene, Gerard, Hill, and the redoubtable Nicholas Culpepper were standard works. *Thomas Tusser's Five Hundred Points of Good Husbandry* was still popular, as was Dr. Andrew Boorde's sixteenth-century *Breviary of Health. The English Housewife* by Gervaise Markham, a seventeenth-century publication, made it clear that this busy lady was expected to have a working knowledge of medicine, cooking, gardening, and distilling.

These useful volumes were brought to the New World by the early colonists along with seeds of culinary and medicinal plants, many of which have become naturalized in America.

Early settlers were plagued by fever, ague, gripings of the belly, smallpox, colds, pleurisies, and empyemas, which took heavy toll during the first years, as well as headaches, palsies, dropsies, worms, scurvies, and toothaches. The latter were very prevalent, an affliction for which Cotton Mather, in his *Angel of Bethesda*, gives no less than eighteen remedies.

"Among the plantes of our soyle" the Reverend Mather quotes Sir William Temple as singling out "five as being of the greatest vertue and most friendly to health: sage, rue, saffron, alehoof, garlick, and elder." "The wonders of sage," Dr. Mather tells us, "can't be reckoned up."

Dr. Mather was not unaware of the writings of Dioscorides, Pliny, and Theophrastus. In a chapter called "The Physick Garden," he mentions them all, as well as the English herbalists.

He extols the use of wild as well as cultivated herbs. "Coltsfoot," he says, "has been found a most potent analeptic." Celandine tea he has heard, "cried up at such a rate, that if half be true 'tis one of the best things in the world."

Mather the minister and theologian speaks between medical recipes. "Christian: the vertues of every plant call for thy praises to the glorious God who has made the plant and taught us the value of it."

XII

Honey and Vinegar

Honey was prescribed as a suitable, and itself curative, vehicle for mixing herbal remedies fifteen thousand years ago. It has been an important part of the pharmacopeia of all nations—Egypt, Assyria, China, Greece, and Rome. In the thirteenth century the Spanish-born, Egyptian-educated Maimonides described a combination of honey and vinegar, predating Vermont's folk doctor, D. C. Jarvis, by seventeen centuries. He called this mixture "oxymel" and asserted that it was good to open obstructions in the liver and spleen, to stimulate a flow of urine and to help the intestines pass excess bile.

The Egyptians were convinced that honey contained a miraculous life substance which could pass on to the person who ate it both purity, power, health, and longevity in this world and, no doubt, protection in the next. Sealed jars of the golden liquid were found in the tombs of the Pharaohs.

These ancient Egyptians knew something which we, after fifteen hundred years, are just rediscovering. Honey has great disinfectant qualities, which modern scientists call "hygroscopic." This means that honey draws every bit of moisture out of germs, and germs, even as human beings, perish without water. Experiments have been made recently which show that some of the most virulent germs can endure only twenty-four to one hundred hours in the sweet fluid which bees manufacture from the nectar of flowers, although they retain their deadly strength forty days and longer if not immersed in honey. Typhoid fever and bronchial pneumonia germs were among the ones tested.

All of this points to some very specific action for those of use who want to stay healthy and to cure our own diseases if we get any. But let us remember that all of the above uses of honey employed only pure, unboiled honey just as it came from the hive, undiluted. We can use this type of honey, available from the nearest apiary or health food store, as a daily sweetener.

We can use honey to mix herbal remedies such as cough syrups, and in disinfectants for exterior and interior infections.

Honey's hygroscopic uses should not be forgotten. Use it to remove eye film. Experiment with it for other uses; remember that this magic amber liquid has a long and honorable history of helping everything from proper growth to vital and enjoyable longevity and that no harm has ever come from its use. It contains, in varying degrees (depending on the soil in which the plants grew from which the bees extracted the nectar): iron, copper, manganese, silica, chlorine, calcium, potassium, sodium, phosphorus, aluminum, and manganese.

The final bonanza of honey is its vitamin content: Vitamin B, thiamine, Vitamin B_2, riboflavin, Vitamin C, ascorbic acid, and pantothenic acid, pyridoxine, and nicotinic acid.

One of the well-known, invisible, battles that goes on in our bodies is between cells and bacteria, a battle over the possession of fluid or moisture. This is not surprising because water has always been, and will always be, the liquid of life. In water life on earth began, and without it it cannot exist. When bacteria invade our bodies, they attempt to sustain themselves by taking moisture from the body cells; but if these cells are not deficient in potassium, they can take the moisture from the invading bacteria. The cells can win this tug of war if we provide them with potassium by eating enough natural foods—fruit, leaves, roots, honey, and vinegar—to turn the moisture-absorbing race in favor of the cells. Vinegar is excellent for this purpose as it combines potassium with phosphorus, chlorine, sodium, magnesium, calcium, sulphur, iron, fluorine, silicon, and many trace minerals.

Apple-cider vinegar can turn the alkaline-acid balance in our bodies in favor of acid which is a preventative against food poisoning. One or two teaspoons of apple-cider vinegar (without preservatives, made from whole apples) in a glass of water, taken twice a day, will maintain a healthy balance in the body. Wine vinegar can be substituted if you cannot get an apple-cider vinegar without preservatives. The custom, in all European countries, of drinking a glass of wine with a meal has the same effect.

Vinegar, added to bath water, will keep the skin healthy and rosy. It stimulates circulation and keeps the pores open. Used as a rinse, it will give the hair a glossy appearance and a soft texture.

APPENDIX I

Alphabetical List of Herbs

Agrimony	*Agrimonia eupatoria*
Aloe	*Aloe vera*
Angelica	*Angelica archangelica*
Anise	*Pimpinella anisum*
Basil	*Ocimum basilicum*
Bearberry	*Arctostaphylos uva-ursi*
Bee Balm	*Monarda didyma*
Boneset	*Eupatorium perfoliatum*
Borage	*Borago officinalis*
Bugle	*Ajuga reptans*
Burdock	*Arctium lappa*
Calendula	*Calendula officinalis*
Caraway	*Carum carvi*

Catnip	*Nepeta cataria*
Cayenne Pepper	*Capsicum frutescens*
Celandine	*Chelidonium majus*
Chamomile	*Chamaemelum mobile*
Chervil	*Anthriscus cerefolium*
Chickweed	*Stellaria media*
Clover	*Trifolium pratense*
Cohosh	*Caulophyllum thalictroides*
Coltsfoot	*Tussilago farfara*
Comfrey	*Symphytum officinale*
Coneflower	*Echinacea angustifolia*
Coriander	*Coriandrum sativum*
Corn	*Zea mays*
Costmary	*Balsamita major*
Couch Grass	*Agropyron repens*
Dandelion	*Taraxacum officinale*
Dill	*Anethum graveolens*
Elder	*Sambucus canadensis*
Elecampane	*Inula helenium*
Evening Primrose	*Oenothera biennis*
Fenugreek	*Trigonella foenum-graecum*
Fennel	*Foeniculum vulgare*
Feverfew	*Tanacetum parthenium*
Fireweed	*Epilobium angustifolium*
Garlic	*Allium sativum*
Ginger	*Asarum canadense*
Goldenrod	*Solidago* species
Goldthread	*Coptis groenlandica*
Ground-Ivy	*Glechoma hederacea*
Hawkweed	*Hieracium pilosella*
Horehound	*Marrubium vulgare*
Horsetail	*Equisetum arvense*
Hyssop	*Hyssopus officinalis*
Jewel Weed	*Impatiens capensis*
Lady's Mantle	*Alchemilla xanthochlora*
Lavender	*Lavandula angustifolia*
Lemon Balm	*Melissa officinalis*
Lovage	*Levisticum officinale*
Mallow	*Malva sylvestris*
Marjoram	*Origanum* species

Meadowsweet	*Filipendula ulmaria*
Milk Thistle	*Silybum marianum*
Milkweed	*Asclepias syriaca*
Mint	*Mentha* species
Mullein	*Verbascum thapsus*
Myrrh	*Commiphora myrrha*
Nettle	*Urtica dioica*
Parsley	*Petroselinum crispum*
Plantain	*Plantago major*
Purslane	*Portulaca oleracea*
Rosemary	*Rosmarinus officinalis*
Rue	*Ruta graveolens*
Sage	*Salvia officinalis*
St. John's-wort	*Hypericum perforatum*
Salad Burnet	*Sanguisorba officinalis*
Savory	*Satureja hortensis*
Self heal	*Prunella vulgaris*
Sorrel	*Rumex* species
Strawberry	*Fragaria virginiana*
Sweet Cicely	*Myrris odorata*
Sweet Woodruff	*Galium odoratum*
Tansy	*Tanacetum vulgare*
Thyme	*Thymus vulgaris*
Valerian	*Valeriana officinalis*
Vervain	*Verbena hastata*
Wintergreen	*Gaultheria procumbens*
Wormwood	*Artemisia absinthium*
Yarrow	*Achillea millefolium*

APPENDIX II

The Language of Herbalists

Like many new vocabularies, the words herbalists use to describe the medicinal actions of herbs are sometimes familiar in ordinary conversation, and sometimes strange. "Aromatic" and "astringent," for example, are general rather than scientific terms. None of the words are so uncommon that they will be found only in medical or scientific journals. "Demulcent" and "emollient" are terms used to describe a quality of soothing bodily tissue. The first refers to the interior of the body, the second to the exterior. "Diaphoretic" and "diuretic" refer to the action of herbs that help the body to remove toxic material, through the sweat glands and through the kidneys.

We use these words to describe the medicinal action of individual herbs because they convey a meaning in one word that would otherwise take from two to seven words to make clear. They are listed here for convenience and easy referral, but many of them you will already know.

Abortifacient: Induces abortion.
Alterative: Non-specific action which improves the general health of the body through stimulation of the functioning of its parts. Should be taken over a long period of time.
Anodyne: Soothes or relieves pain.
Anthelmintic: Dispels or destroys intestinal worms.
Antibiotic: Destroys micro-organisms in the body.
Antiperiodic: Prevents recurrence of a disease.
Antirheumatic: Prevents rheumatism or relieves its symptoms.
Antiscorbutic: Source of Vitamin C, prevents scurvy.
Antiscrofulous: Prevents scrofula.
Antiseptic: Destroys and/or inhibits harmful bacteria.
Antispasmodic: Relieves and/or stops spasms and cramps.
Aperient: Acts as a mild laxative.
Aromatic: Has a pleasant and stimulating scent.
Astringent: Contracts tissue, reduces body secretions.
Carminative: Expels gas from the intestines.
Chologogue: Increases the flow of bile into the intestines.
Coagulant: Increases the clotting of blood.
Condiment: Acts as a strong seasoning, enhancing the flavor of foods.
Demulcent: Soothes irritated tissue and mucous membrane in the body.
Deobstruent: Opens natural passages of the body.
Diaphoretic: Promotes involuntary perspiration.
Diuretic: Increases secretion and flow of urine.
Emetic: Causes vomiting.
Emmenagogue: Promotes menstrual flow.
Emollient: Softens and soothes the skin.
Expectorant: Causes discharge of mucus from respiratory system.
Febrifuge: Reduces fever.
Galactagogue: Increases secretion of milk.
Hemostatic: Stops bleeding.
Hepatic: Acts on the liver.
Laxative: A mild purgative.
Lithostyptic: Good for disposing of kidney stones.
Mucilaginous: Has gummy or gelatinous consistency.
Nervine: Has a soothing effect on the nerves.
Parturient: Aids childbirth.

Pectoral: Remedies pulmonary disease.
Purgative: Causes thorough emptying of the bowels.
Refrigerant: Lowers body heat.
Rubefacient: Produces mild local irritation and redness of the skin.
Sedative: Soothes the nerves, relieves tension.
Stimulant: Temporarily quickens a vital process of the body.
Styptic: Checks bleeding.
Stomachic: Stimulates gastric digestion.
Tonic: Invigorates and strengthens the entire body.
Vermifuge: Expels intestinal worms.
Vulnerary: Heals wounds.

APPENDIX III

List of Vitamins and Their Effects

Vitamin A: Promotes normal vision, prevents night blindness, promotes smooth skin, can prevent formation of cells that later may turn into cancer cells. It also protects epithelial tissue.

Vitamin B_1: Thiamine is necessary for the body to make proper use of carbohydrates.

Vitamin B_2: Riboflavin is needed to enable the stomach to secrete enough digestive juices to absorb the nutrients that are put into it. Lack of B_2 can cause adverse skin and mouth conditions and eye fatigue.

Vitamin B_3: Niacin prevents pellagra and has been used in treating migraine headaches and to relieve arthritis pains.

Vitamin B_6: Pyridoxine soothes the nerves. It has been used by women during pregnancy. It helps the body assimilate proteins.

Pantothenic acid: Essential for cell growth. It delays body changes due to increased age. Deficiency in pantothenic acid can impair the function of the adrenal glands which may cause inability to deal with stress, muscle weakness, and the sensation of "pins and needles" in hands and legs.

Inositol: The essential growth factor. It keeps the arteries from clogging thereby preventing high blood pressure.

Biotin: Keeps energy high and improves mental health during the later years of life.

Choline: Promotes health of the liver and aids the function of the gall bladder.

Vitamin B_{12}: Necessary in the formation of hemoglobin, the coloring matter in the red blood corpuscles which brings oxygen to the body tissues. Prevents pellagra and pernicious anemia.

Vitamin B_{15}: Pangamic acid supplies oxygen to the body cells and the heart. Acts as a detoxicant. It has been used to treat heart trouble, emphysema, and premature aging.

Folic acid: Prevents anemia. Like B_{12} it is needed for production of normal red blood cells.

PABA (para-amino-benzoic acid): A part of folic acid. Promotes skin health and is thought to prevent and restore gray hair.

Vitamin C: Maintains healthy connective tissue in the body, protects the walls of the blood vessels, and overcomes infections.

Vitamin D: Essential to the metabolism of calcium and phosphorus and to proper growth.

Vitamin E: Tocopherol is necessary for growth and the function of the reproductive glands and organs. It strengthens heart muscles, repairs and strengthens cells and repairs scar tissue.

Vitamin F: Includes arachidonic, linoleic, and other oleic acids. These acids are valuable for two reasons. They have nutritive value in themselves and they contain open links, or double bands, in their chains which enable them to absorb the molecules that the body wishes to have transported to wherever cell-building is taking place.

Vitamin K: Tyrosinase catalyzes the aerobic oxidation of tyrosine into melanin and other pigments. It is necessary for blood coagulation.

Vitamin P: Rutin is essential for healthy veins and arteries and normal blood pressure. It can help in the prevention of strokes.

Vitamin U: Thought to act on ulcers in a curative way, Vitamin U is found in raw cabbage, and has also been identified in celery, raw milk, and uncooked greens.

APPENDIX IV

Sources of Herb Seeds and Plants

W. Atlee Burpee Company, Warminster, PA 18974.

Capriland Herb Farm, Silver St., Coventry, CT 06238.

Comstock Ferre and Company, 263 Main St., Wethersfield, CT 06109.

The Cook's Garden, P.O. Box 65, Londonderry, VT 05148.

Fedco Seeds, 52 Mayflowerhill Dr., Waterville, ME 04301.

The Herb Cottage, Washington Cathedral, Mount Saint Alban, Washington, DC.

Le Jardin du Gourmet (Raymond Saufroy Imports), West Danville, VT 05873.

Logee's Greenhouses, 55 North St., Danielson, CT 06239.

Meadowbrook Herb Gardens, Wyoming, RI 02898.

Nichols Garden Nursery, 1190 North Pacific Highway, Albany, OR 97321.

George W. Park Seed Company, Greenwood, SC 29647.

Pine Tree Garden Seeds, New Gloucester, ME 04260.
Seed Savers' Exchange (Kent Whealy, Director), Rural Route 3, Box 239, Decorah, IA 52101.
Thompson and Morgan, P.O. Box 1308, Jackson, NJ 08527.

SOURCES FOR BOTANICALS*

Geological Botany Company, 622 West 67th St., Kansas City, MO 64113.
The Herb Shop, Box 352, Orem, UT 84601.
Indiana Botanic Gardens, Inc., Box 5, Hammond, IN 46325.
Kiehl Pharmacy, 109 Third Ave., New York, NY 10003.
Wide World of Herbs, 11 St. Catherine St., East, Montreal, Canada H24 1K3.

* Dried herbs and herbal preparations.

Bibliography

SELECT LIST OF HERBALS

Abner, Agnes. *Herbals—Their Origin and Evolution, A Chapter in the History of Botany.* London: Cambridge University Press, 1955 (reprinted 1988).

Bethel, May. *The Healing Power of Herbs.* North Hollywood: Wilshire Book Company, 1974.

Boorde, Andrew. *The Breviary of Health.* London: Thomas East, 1546.

Clymer, R. Swinburne. *Nature's Healing Agents.* Quakertown, Pa.: The Humanitarian Society, 1973.

Coles, William. *The Art of Simpling.* Limited edition printed from the 1657 edition. Falls Village, Conn.: The Herb Grower Press, 1938.

Culpepper, Nicholas. *Culpepper's Complete Herbal.* London: W. Foulsham and Company, Ltd., 1955. From original edition of 1650.

De la Cruz, Martin, and Juannes Badianus. *The Badianus Manuscript, an Aztec Herbal of 1552.* Edited by Emily Walcott Emmart. Baltimore: The Johns Hopkins Press, 1940.

Dioscorides, Pedanius, of Anazarbos. *De materia medica.* Edited and first printed by Robert T. Gunther, 1933. Facsimile edition, New York and London: Hafner Publishing Company, 1968.

Evelyn, John. *Acetaria, A Discourse of Sallets.* London: D. Toose, 1699, 1706. Reprint, Brooklyn: Brooklyn Botanic Garden, 1937.

———. *The Kalendarium Hortense or the Gardener's Almanac,* 10th Edition (1706). Reprint, Falls Village, Conn.: The Herb Grower Press, 1963.

Fuchs, Leonhart. *De historia stirpium.* Basle: Isingrin Press, 1542.

Gerard, John. *The Herball or General Historie of Plantes, Gathered by John Gerard of London, Master in Chirurgerie, Very Much Enlarged and Amended by Thomas Johnson, Citizen, an Apothecarye of London.* London: Adam, Islip, Joice Norton and Richard Whitakers, 1633.

Greene, William. *The Universal Herbal.* London: Coxton Press, 1816, 1824.

Grieve, Maude. *A Modern Herball.* 2 volumes. New York and London: Hafner Publishing Company, 1931, 1955, 1967. New York: Harcourt, Brace, and Company, 1931. New York: Dover Publications, 1971.

Leyel, C. F. *The Truth About Herbs.* London: Andrew Dakers, Ltd., 1934.

Lust, John B. *The Herb Book.* New York: Bantam Books, 1974.

Meydenback, Jacob. *Gart der Gesundheit.* Mainz, 1485.

———. *Hortus Sanitatis.* Mainz, 1491.

Monardes, Nicholas. *Dos Libros.* Seville: Hernando Diaz, 1569.

———. *Joyfull newes out of the newe founde worlde . . .* Translated by John Frampton, Marchaunt. London: W. Norton, 1577.

Parkinson, John. *Paradisi in Sole, Paradisus Terrestris.* Faithfully reprinted from the edition of 1629. London: Methuen and Company, 1904.

Theophrastus. *Enquiry into plants and minor works on odours and weather signs.* English translation by Sir Arthur Hort. Cambridge, Mass.: Harvard University Press, 1949.

Thompson, Campbell. *Assyrian Herbal, A Monograph on Assyrian Vegetable Drugs.* London, 1924.

Turner, William. *Libellus de Re Herbaria* (1538) and *The Names of Herbs* (1548). Facsimile, London: The Ray Society, 1965.

Veith, Ilza. *The Yellow Emperor's Classic of Internal Medicine. (Hung Ti Nei Chung Su Wen).* Chapters 1–34 translated from the Chinese with an introductory study. Berkeley: University of California Press, 1966.

Weiner, Michael A. *Earth Medicine, Earth Foods.* New York: The Macmillan Company, 1972.

HISTORICAL BIBLIOGRAPHY

Brown, Alice Cooke. *Medicinal Plants and Their History*. New York: Bonanza Books, 1966.

Campbell, Donald. *Arabian Medicine and Its Influence on the Middle Ages*. London: Kegan, Paul, Trench, Trubner and Company Ltd., 1926.

Freeman, Margaret B. *Herbs of the Medieval Household, for Cooking, Healing, and Divers Uses*. New York: Metropolitan Museum of Art, 1943.

Hartman, Franz. *The Life and Doctrines of Phillipus Theophrastus, Bombast of Hohenheim, Known by the Name of Paracelsus*. New York: The Metaphysical Publishers Company, 1891.

Jeffers, Robert H. *The Friends of John Gerard (1545–1612) Surgeon and Botanist*. Falls Village, Conn.: The Herb Grower Press, 1975.

Larson, William. *The Country House-Wives' Garden*. London: Anne Grifflen, 1637.

Lockwood, Alice G. B., editor. *Gardens of Colony and State: Gardens and Gardeners of the American Colonies and the Republic Before 1840*. New York: Charles Scribners Sons, 1931, 1934.

Pagel, Walter. *Paracelsus—An Introduction to Philosophical Medicine in the Era of the Renaissance*. Basel and New York: S. Karger, 1958.

Rohde, Eleanor Sinclair. *The Olde English Herbals*. London, New York: Longmans, Green and Company, 1922. New York: Dover Publications, 1971.

MEDICINAL BIBLIOGRAPHY

Baas, John Hermann. *Outline of the History of Medicine and the Medical Profession*. Translated, and in conjunction with the author revised and enlarged by H. E. Henderson. New York: J. H. Vail and Company, 1889.

Clymer, R. Swinburne. *Nature's Healing Agents*. Quakertown, Pa.: The Humanitarian Society, 1973.

Goodman, Louis S., and Alfred Gilman. *The Pharmacological Basis of Therapeutics*, 4th Edition. London: The Macmillan Company, 1970.

Harrison, Tinsley Randolph. *Harrison's Principles of Internal Medicine*, 7th Edition. New York: McGraw Hill Book Company, 1974.

Jarvis, D. C. *Folk Medicine*. New York: Holt, Rhinehart and Winston, 1958. Greenwich, Conn.: Fawcett Publications, 1973.

Jefferson, R. *The Family Doctor: A Dictionary of Domestic Medicine and Surgery Especially Adapted for Family Use*, 15th Edition. Philadelphia: George Gebbie, Publisher, 1869.

Kloss, Jethro. *Back to Eden.* Coalmont, Tenn.: Longview Publishing House, 1971.

Kreig, Margaret B. *Green Medicine.* New York: Rand McNally and Company, 1964.

Krochmal, Arnold, and Connie Krochmal. *A Guide to the Medicinal Plants of the United States.* New York: Quadrangle Books, 1973.

Marks, Geoffrey, and William K. Beatty. *The Story of Medicine in America.* New York: Charles Scribner's Sons, 1973.

Maimonides, Moses. *Medical Aphorisms.* Translated and edited by Fred Rosner and Munther Suessman. New York: Yeshiva University Press, 1971.

Mather, Cotton. *The Angel of Bethesda.* Edited, with an introduction and notes by Gordon W. Jones. Barre, Mass.: American Antiquarian Society and Barre Publishers, 1972.

Millspaugh, Charles F. *American Medicinal Plants 1892.* New York: Yeshiva University Press, 1971. New York: Dover Publications, 1974.

Pierce, R. V. *The People's Common Sense Medical Advisor in Plain English: Or, Medicine Simplified,* 42nd Edition. Buffalo, N.Y.: World Dispensary Printing Office, 1895.

Thomson, Samuel. *Thomsonian Materia Medica, or Botanic Family Physician.* Albany, N.Y.: J. Munsell, 1841, 1847.

Trease, George. *A Text Book of Pharmacognasy.* London: Balliere, Tindale and Cassell, 1966.

Vogel, Virgil J. *American Indian Medicine.* Norman: University of Oklahoma Press, 1970.

Wheelwright, Edith Grey. *Medicinal Plants and Their History.* New York: Dover Publications, 1974.

Wren, R. W., editor. *Potter's New Cyclopedia of Medicinal Herbs and Preparations.* New York: Harper and Row, 1972; 8th ed. 1989.

Youngken, Herber W. *Pharmaceutical Botany.* Philadelphia: The Blakiston Company, 1951.

SUGGESTED READINGS

Botanical

Britton, Nathaniel, and Addison Brown. *An Illustrated Flora of the Northern United States and Canada.* New York: Dover Publications, 1970.

Foster, Steven, and James A. Duke. *Peterson Field Guides: Eastern/Central Medicinal Plants.* Boston: Houghton Mifflin Company, 1990.

Peterson, Roger Tory, and Margaret McKenny. *A Field Guide to Wildflowers of Northeastern and North-Central North America.* Boston: Houghton Mifflin Company, 1968.

Folklore

Jacob, Dorothy. *A Witch's Guide to Gardening.* New York: Taplinger Publishing Company, 1965.

Lehner, Ernst, and Johanna Lehner. *Folklore and Symbolism of Flowers, Plants and Trees.* New York: Tudor Publishing Company, 1960.

Lucas, E. H. *Folklore and Plant Drugs.* Papers of the Michigan Academy of Science, Arts and Letters, Vol. XLV, 1960.

Meyer, Clarence. *American Folk Medicine.* New York: Thomas Y. Crowell Company, 1973.

Oldmeadow, Katherine I. *The Folklore of Herbs.* Birmingham: Cornish Brothers, 1946.

General (History, Culinary, Gardens)

Beston, Henry. *Herbs and the Earth.* Garden City, N.Y.: Doubleday, Doran and Company, 1935.

Burlington Ecumenical Action Ministry. *The Home Health Handbook.* Brattleboro: The Stephen Greene Press, 1972.

Burroughs, John. *A Year in the Fields.* Boston: Houghton, Mifflin and Company, 1901.

Crow, W. B. *The Occult Properties of Herbs.* London: Aquarian Press, 1969.

Mességué, Maurice. *Of People and Plants.* Rochester, VT.: Healing Arts Press, 1991.

Sanecki, Kay N. *The Complete Book of Herbs.* New York: The Macmillan Publishing Company, 1974.

The School of Salernum. *Regimen Sanitatis Salerni.* Salerno: Provinciale per il Turismo, 1957.

Tompkins, Peter, and Christopher Bird. *The Secret Life of Plants.* New York: Harper and Row, 1973.

Health

Adams, Ruth. *The Complete Home Guide to all the Vitamins.* New York: Larchmont Books, 1975.

Hall, Ross Hume. *Food for Naught.* New York: Random House, 1976.

Hunter, Beatrice Trum. *The Great Nutrition Robbery.* New York: Charles Scribner's Sons, 1978.

The Staff of *Prevention* Magazine. *The Encyclopedia of Common Diseases.* Emmaus, Pa.: The Rodale Press, 1976.

Herb Gardening

Foster, Gertrude. *Herbs for Every Garden.* New York: E. P. Dutton, 1973.

Handbook of Herbs #27. Brooklyn: Brooklyn Botanic Garden, no date.

Kamm, Minnie W. *Old Time Herbs for Northern Gardens.* New York: Dover Publications, 1971.

Philbrick, Helen, and Richard Gregg. *Companion Plants and How to Use Them.* Old Greenwich, Conn.: The Devin–Adair Company, 1966, 1971, 1973.

Simmons, Adelma Grenier. *Herb Gardening in Five Seasons.* New York: Hawthorne Books, 1971.

———. *Herb Gardens of Delight.* New York: Hawthorne Books, 1974.

———. *The Illustrated Herbal Handbook.* New York: Hawthorne Books, 1972.

Smith A. W. *A Gardener's Book of Plant Names.* New York: Harper & Row, 1963.

Periodicals

The Herb Grower Magazine. Falls Village, Conn. 06031. A quarterly devoted to herb gardening.

Organic Gardening and Farming. 33 East Minor St., Emmaus, Pa. 18049. A monthly devoted to organic gardening and living. Contains frequent articles on herbs.

Prevention. 33 East Minor St., Emmaus, Pa. 18049. A monthly devoted to maintaining good health.

Index

Partridgeberry, 210–11 *(ill., 210)*
Pendulum, 222
Pennyroyal, 69, 72, 73
Peppermint, 72, 94
Perspiration, 59, 67, 69, 211
Pesto (recipe), 37, 79
Pewterwurt, 144–5 *(ill., 144)*
Pimples, 107, 138
Pineapple sage, 81–2 *(ill., 81)*
Pineapple weed, 47
Plantain, 163–4 *(ill., 163)*
Pleurisy, 199
Pleurisy root, 69
Poison ivy, 38, 62
Potato soup (recipe), 47
Poultice, 27
Primrose (evening), 130 *(ill., 131)*
Prostate problems, 230
Psoriasis, 188
Purslane, 164–5 *(ill., 165)*

Quack grass, 123–5 *(ill., 124)*

Raspberry, 240
Recipes:
  basil pesto, 37
  candied angelica, 109
  carob mint pudding, 95
  claret cup, 153
  crème de menthe, 95
  dandelion wine, 100–1
  eggs beurre noir, 22
  elderberry jelly, 130
  elderberry wines, 129
  herb jellies, 99
  herb vinegars, 100
  horehound candy, 43
  Kahlua, 154
  lime sherbert, 98
  marinade for pork, 59–60
  minted carrots, 94–5
  oil of garlic, 137–8
  parsley butter, 79

  potato soup, 47
  salad dressing, 94
  sorrel soup, 172
  summer soup, 97
  Swedish meatballs, 180
  Tansy, 176–8
  tempura, 34–5
  vegetable casserole, 75
  whole wheat biscuits, 34
  zucchini pancakes, 98
Remedies. *See* Herbal remedies;
  Tea
Respiratory ailments, 59, 109, 137,
  155, 156, 162, 206, 217
Rheumatism, 69, 75, 78, 88, 116,
  133, 138, 147, 149, 156, 164,
  166, 182, 189, 202, 211
Rhizome, 11, 13, 25 *(ill., 12)*
Ribwort, 163–4 *(ill., 163)*
Rickets, 234
Root, 11 *(ill., 12)*
  collecting, 25
  drying, 102–3
Rosemary, 166–8, 190, 243
  (ill., 167)
Rue, 168–70 *(ill., 169)*
Rupture, 145

Sage, 38, 79–82 *(ill., 80)*
St. John's wort, 206–8 *(ill., 207)*
Salad, 94, 201
  dressing, 94
  greens, 34, 36, 55, 64, 78, 84,
   111, 164, 172, 225
Salad burnet, 36, 83–4 *(ill., 83)*
Salves, 128, 164, 189
  basic procedure, 27, 188–9
Savory, 84–6 *(ill., 85)*
Sciatica, 75, 78, 107, 128, 139, 168,
  176, 179, 206, 211, 232, 234
Seeds:
  drying, 103
Self-heal, 170–1 *(ill., 171)*